Posttraumatic and Acute Stress Disorders

Fifth Edition

Matthew J. Friedman, MD, PhD

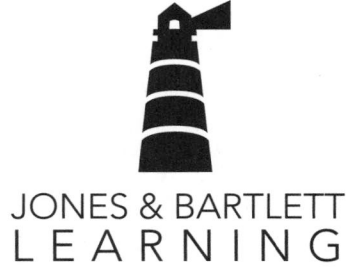

JONES & BARTLETT
LEARNING

World Headquarters

Jones & Bartlett Learning
40 Tall Pine Drive
Sudbury, MA 01776
978-443-5000
info@jblearning.com
www.jblearning.com

Jones & Bartlett Learning Canada
6339 Ormindale Way
Mississauga, Ontario L5V 1J2
Canada

Jones & Bartlett Learning International
Barb House, Barb Mews
London W6 7PA
United Kingdom

Jones & Bartlett Learning books and products are available through most bookstores and online booksellers. To contact Jones & Bartlett Learning directly, call 800-832-0034, fax 978-443-8000, or visit our website, www.jblearning.com.

Substantial discounts on bulk quantities of Jones & Bartlett Learning publications are available to corporations, professional associations, and other qualified organizations. For details and specific discount information, contact the special sales department at Jones & Bartlett Learning via the above contact information or send an email to specialsales@jblearning.com.

The authors, editor, and publisher have made every effort to provide accurate information. However, they are not responsible for errors, omissions, or for any outcomes related to the use of the contents of this book and take no responsibility for the use of the products and procedures described. Treatments and side effects described in this book may not be applicable to all people; likewise, some people may require a dose or experience a side effect that is not described herein. Drugs and medical devices are discussed that may have limited availability controlled by the Food and Drug Administration (FDA) for use only in a research study or clinical trial. Research, clinical practice, and government regulations often change the accepted standard in this field. When consideration is being given to use of any drug in the clinical setting, the healthcare provider or reader is responsible for determining FDA status of the drug, reading the package insert, and reviewing prescribing information for the most up-to-date recommendations on dose, precautions, and contraindications, and determining the appropriate usage for the product. This is especially important in the case of drugs that are new or seldom used.

Production Credits

Executive Publisher: Christopher Davis
Editorial Assistant: Sara Cameron
Production Director: Amy Rose
Production Editor: Daniel Stone
Associate Marketing Manager: Katie Hennessy
V.P., Manufacturing and Inventory Control:
    Therese Connell

Project Management: Thistle Hill Publishing
    Services, LLC
Composition: Dedicated Business Solutions, Inc.
Cover Design: Scott Moden
Cover Image: © Robert O. Brown Photography/
    ShutterStock, Inc.
Printing and Binding: Malloy, Incorporated
Cover Printing: Malloy, Incorporated

Library of Congress Cataloging-in-Publication Data

Friedman, Matthew J.
  Posttraumatic and acute stress disorders / Matthew J. Friedman. — 5th ed.
    p. ; cm.
  Rev. ed. of: Post-traumatic and acute stress disorders / by Matthew Friedman. 4th ed. Kansas City, MO : Compact Clinicals, c2006.
  Includes bibliographical references and index.
  ISBN-13: 978-0-7637-9568-9 (pbk.)
  ISBN-10: 0-7637-9568-2 (pbk.)
  1. Post-traumatic stress disorder. 2. Post-traumatic stress disorder—Treatment. I. Friedman, Matthew J. Post-traumatic and acute stress disorders. II. Title.
  [DNLM: 1. Stress Disorders, Post-Traumatic—diagnosis. 2. Stress Disorders, Post-Traumatic—psychology. 3. Stress Disorders, Post-Traumatic—therapy. WM 172]
  RC552.P67F749 2012
  616.85'2106—dc22
                  2010040259

6048

Printed in the United States of America
14 13 12 11 10   10 9 8 7 6 5 4 3 2 1

Contents

Chapter 4: Psychological Treatments for PTSD

Chapter 5: Pharmacological Treatments for PTSD

Chapter 6: Strategies for Acute Stress Reactions and Acute Stress Disorder (ASD)

Chapter 1
Overview of Posttraumatic Stress Disorder (PTSD)

This chapter answers the following questions:

- ▶ **What Is Trauma?**—This section defines trauma, the necessary precursor to PTSD.
- ▶ **What Is the History and Prevalence of PTSD?**—This section reviews how PTSD has been viewed since ancient times and presents information on how common PTSD is worldwide.
- ▶ **Can PTSD Be Prevented?**—This section offers recommendations for promoting resilience among those at risk for PTSD.
- ▶ **How Severe and Chronic Is PTSD?**—This section identifies three general categories of PTSD sufferers: those with lifetime PTSD, those in remission but experiencing occasional relapses, and those with delayed onset.

DURING the course of a lifetime, everyone is exposed to stressful events such as failure, disappointment, rejection, and loss. Most of the time, most of us have the psychological capacity to cope successfully with such events and to continue our lives pretty much as before. Sometimes we are confronted by terrifying, catastrophic, or severely stressful (e.g., "traumatic") events in which there is a real possibility that we and/or a loved one might be killed or seriously injured. As with less stressful events, most of us are resilient and will bounce back from the fear, helplessness, or horror that we experienced during the traumatic event. A significant minority of us, however, will be unable to cope psychologically with such traumatic stress. We will not bounce back but, instead, will develop the serious, and potentially incapacitating, symptoms that characterize PTSD.

In the United States, approximately half of all Americans will be exposed to at least one traumatic event, such as assault, military combat, an industrial or vehicular accident, rape, domestic violence, or a natural disaster (e.g., an earthquake). Traumatic exposure is higher for individuals who engage in professions where their work places them in traumatic situations on a regular basis; this includes military personnel, police, firefighters, emergency medical technicians, and others. Exposure to extreme stress is also much higher for people who live in nations subjected to war, state terrorism, or forced migration, such as Algeria, Cambodia, Palestine, or Iraq. As stated previously, most people can absorb the psychological impact of such experiences and resume their normal lives; however, a sizeable number cannot.

Approximately 8 percent of Americans and 20 to 30 percent elsewhere (in areas of conflict) will suffer from PTSD.[1,2]

PTSD was first defined as a distinct psychiatric diagnosis in 1980 when the American Psychiatric Association published its revised diagnostic manual, the Diagnostic and Statistical Manual of Mental Disorders—Third Edition (DSM–III).[3]

The term *posttraumatic stress disorder (PTSD)* describes the condition a person experiences when trauma-related symptoms or impairments in everyday functioning last for at least a month and sometimes for life. PTSD has been recognized by many other names since antiquity and by modern psychiatry since the late 1800s. Although the specific symptoms included in the original PTSD diagnostic criteria have been partially modified, the fundamental PTSD construct has clearly withstood the test of time. As a result, clinicians have had 30 years in which to utilize PTSD as a diagnostic tool and to develop effective treatments.

Although PTSD can only be diagnosed one month after an individual has been exposed to trauma, many people experience great distress during the immediate aftermath of a traumatic event, including having nightmares and avoiding people and places that may remind them of the trauma. Such acute, posttraumatic reactions will be considered in Chapter 6.

What Is Trauma?

For a list of the specific diagnostic criteria for PTSD, see page 12.

When "trauma" was first introduced as a construct in the *DSM–III* diagnostic criteria for PTSD, it was defined as a catastrophic stressor that "would evoke significant symptoms of distress in most people."[3] Trauma was thought to be a rare and overwhelming event—"generally outside the range of usual human experience"—that differed qualitatively from "common experiences, such as: bereavement, chronic illness, business losses, or marital conflict." Traumatic events cited in *DSM–III* included rape, assault, torture, incarceration in a death camp, military combat, natural disasters, industrial/vehicular accidents, or exposure to war/civil/domestic violence.

Initially, it was thought that trauma could be defined exclusively in terms of catastrophic events that happened to an individual who was in the wrong place at the wrong time. As initially conceptualized, anyone who had been exposed to war, rape, torture, or natural disaster had been "traumatized."[3] This was changed in the 1994 *DSM–IV* (and retained in the 2000 *DSM–IV–TR*) because it had become apparent that most people exposed to catastrophic events did not develop PTSD.[4,5]

Although exposure to catastrophic stress is a necessary condition, it is not sufficient by itself to "traumatize" an individual. What also matters is the emotional response of the person exposed to such an event. If the rape or accident produced an intense emotional response (characterized in *DSM–IV–TR* as "fear, helplessness, or horror"), the event is "traumatic." If an intense emotional response is not experienced, then the event is not considered a "traumatic event"; therefore, by *DSM* definition, the event cannot cause PTSD.

Today, our understanding about trauma has changed significantly from that first described in the *DSM–III*, essentially focusing on the realizations that:

▶ **Catastrophic events are not rare.** Research has shown that over half of all American men (60.7 percent) and women (51.2 percent) are likely to be exposed to at least one catastrophic event during their lives.[1] Exposure is much higher in countries torn by war, civil strife, genocide, state-sponsored terrorism, or other forms of violence. For example, exposure to trauma was reportedly as high as 92 percent in Algeria, where deadly conflict and violence have persisted for years.[2]

▶ **Trauma is not just an external event.** The concept of trauma has changed from being considered a rare external event (*DSM–III*) to an individual's psychological response to a not-uncommon, overwhelming event (*DSM–IV*). Only people who respond to catastrophic events with fear, helplessness, or horror have been "traumatized" as defined in *DSM–IV–TR*.

> *From a global perspective, exposure to catastrophic stress is a common fact of life.*
>
> *Fifty-four percent of American women who were raped did not develop PTSD; 91 percent of American women involved in an accident did not develop PTSD.[1]*

What Is the History and Prevalence of PTSD?

Historically, poets and writers have recognized that exposure to trauma may produce enduring psychological consequences. Various literary works—Homer's *Iliad*, Shakespeare's *Henry IV*, Dickens's *Tale of Two Cities*—present characters' psychological transformations and symptoms related to trauma. Even Harry Potter was perhaps traumatized when, as an infant, he witnessed his parents' murder by the evil wizard, Lord Voldemort.[6]

From the Patient's Perspective

That lawyer called again. He thinks I've got a great case against the trucking company and could win a huge settlement. It's tempting. I certainly need the money. But every time I even think about the accident (like now), I go to pieces. And—if I start to talk about it, I get terrified. Then the nightmares. No sleep. That horrible jumpy feeling. And I turn into a nervous wreck. It isn't worth it, even if I could win a million bucks! I'll just have to call him back tomorrow and tell him I'm not interested. He'll have to find someone else to sue.

Historical Overview

In the late 19th century, clinicians also began to focus on the psychological impact of military combat among veterans of the U.S. Civil War and the Franco-Prussian War. Clinical formulations on both sides of the Atlantic focused either on cardiovascular (e.g., soldier's heart, Da Costa's syndrome, neurocirculatory asthenia) or psychiatric (e.g., nostalgia, shell shock, combat fatigue, war neurosis) symptoms.[7,8] Similar clinical presentations among 19th-century civilian survivors of train accidents were called "Railway Spine."[9] Throughout this period, clinicians asked to provide treatment for survivors of military or civilian trauma were struck by the physiological as well as the psychological symptoms exhibited. Indeed, by the 1940s, Abram Kardiner, an American psychiatrist who worked extensively with World War I veterans suffering from "War Neurosis," was so impressed by their excessive startle reactions that he called it a "*physioneurosis*."[10]

Prevalence

With the growing recognition that catastrophic stress and traumatic events are much more common than originally suspected, it is clear that PTSD is a significant public health problem. Although over half of all American adults will have been exposed to a catastrophic stress event (60 percent men and 51 percent women), only 6.8–7.8 percent (5 percent men and 10 percent women) will have developed PTSD at some point in their lives.[1] This means that millions of Americans will suffer from this disorder, and PTSD is a major public health problem in the United States and elsewhere. If untreated, many of these individuals will never recover. Research with veterans of World War II and survivors of the Nazi Holocaust has shown, for example, that PTSD can persist for more than 50 years or for a lifetime.[11]

Worldwide, the psychological and physical consequences of traumatic exposure constitute a major public health challenge.[12,13] The long-term impacts of major natural disasters such as the earthquakes in Haiti and Chile, the tsunamis in Indonesia, Sri Lanka, and Thailand, and hurricanes in the south coastal United States can be overwhelming, both for survivors and for aid workers. Countless individuals will be exposed to trauma from war in nations such as Iraq, Afghanistan, and Rwanda as well as Algeria, Palestine, and Bosnia.[14] We must also consider the millions of children and adults exposed to sexual, physical, domestic, criminal, urban, terrorist, and genocidal violence. From this perspective, it is very important to search for effective psychological preventions and to consider providing them to children and adults as part of a global public health strategy.

Chapter 5 reviews some of the major biological abnormalities that are central to this disorder.

physioneurosis—a label for the clinically significant physiological as well as psychological changes believed to be part of the "war neurosis" syndrome

Can PTSD Be Prevented?

Theoretically most PTSD can be prevented. All we have to do is prevent war, rape, interpersonal violence, child abuse, torture, and the like. Although we may all dream of such a utopian state of affairs, it is unlikely to materialize within the foreseeable future. It is also unlikely that natural disasters will ever disappear or that industrial or vehicular accidents will cease to occur. Although many humanitarian and advocacy groups are working to reduce the frequency and toxicity of man-made trauma, primary prevention of PTSD is virtually impossible at this time.

Given the impossibility of successfully preventing traumatic events, the next best approach would be to promote *resilience*—to foster psychobiological attributes and behavioral strategies that will give individuals exposed to trauma the tools they need to cope more effectively with severely stressful situations. Resilience may be promoted at the societal, community, family, and individual levels. Since epidemiologic research consistently indicates that people differ in their vulnerability to (or resilience against) posttraumatic distress, public mental health strategies need to be supported that identify and promote resilience among those at greatest risk for such severe, chronic, and debilitating events:

- ▶ **At the societal level,** developing laws, policies, and practices that ensure optimal preparation for and public responses to large-scale traumatic events such as terrorist attacks and natural disasters
- ▶ **At the community level,** perhaps the most effective psychological strategy for most children and adults would be proactive psychoeducation provided in school, workplace, and community settings
- ▶ **At the family level,** fostering cohesion and mutual support to help the family unit buffer the impact of traumatic stress on its individual members
- ▶ **At the individual level,** enhancing the capacity of individuals to cope with traumatic stress through adaptive strategies, such as protective behaviors, control of physiological responses, or actively seeking social support [15]

If trauma occurs and resilience is insufficient, effective treatment becomes necessary. A number of effective psychosocial and pharmacological treatments have been developed for people with PTSD. This has been a major focus of research in recent years and will be discussed in detail in subsequent chapters (Chapter 4, psychosocial and Chapter 5, pharmacological treatments). Several clinical practice guidelines have evaluated the relative efficacy of such treatment and those evaluations will also be discussed. Finally, some clinical investigators have focused their efforts on developing interventions that might be administered shortly after an individual has been exposed to a traumatic event, with the goal of preventing the later development of PTSD. Such potentially prophylactic approaches will be addressed in Chapter 6.

How Severe and Chronic Is PTSD?

PTSD is no different from other medical or psychiatric disorders in that its severity may range from mild to severe. As with diabetes, heart disease, and depression, some people with PTSD can lead full and rewarding lives despite the disorder. Although there are no current statistics, it appears that a significant minority of patients may develop a persistent, incapacitating mental illness marked by severe and intolerable symptoms; marital, social, and vocational disability; and extensive use of psychiatric and community services. Such people can typically be found on the fringes of society, in homeless shelters, or enrolled in public-sector programs designed for people with persistent mental illnesses, such as *schizophrenia,* from which they are superficially indistinguishable as having PTSD.[16]

The long-term course for most people with chronic PTSD is marked by remissions and relapses. Some people make a full recovery, others partial improvement, and others never improve. Our expectation, of course, is that with the development of effective treatments for people with PTSD (or for preventing the development of PTSD among recently traumatized individuals) we can significantly reduce the prevalence of chronic PTSD.

There are three general classes of PTSD sufferers:

1. **Lifetime PTSD**—Current surveys indicate that 40 percent of patients with *lifetime PTSD* are unlikely to recover whether or not they have ever received treatment.[1] Some may show some improvement in functional capacity or symptom severity, but their PTSD remains chronic, severe, and permanent. It should be understood, however, that effective treatments were not generally available when this survey was conducted.

2. **PTSD in Remission with Occasional Relapses—** Patients in remission, who have been without symptoms for some time, may suddenly relapse and begin to exhibit the full pattern of PTSD symptoms. When this occurs, it is likely that they were recently exposed to a traumatic reminder or some situation that resembled the original traumatic event in a significant way.

3. **Delayed Onset**—In the delayed variant of PTSD, individuals exposed to a traumatic event do not exhibit the

schizophrenia—a major psychiatric disorder characterized by disorganization and fragmentation of thought, delusions, hallucinations, apathy, disturbance of language and communication, and withdrawal from social interaction

lifetime PTSD—those who developed PTSD at any time in their lives

PTSD syndrome until months or years later. As with relapse, the immediate precipitant is usually a situation that resembles the original trauma in a significant way; for example, an American Vietnam veteran whose child has been suddenly deployed to the war zone in Afghanistan or Iraq. On close inspection, most individuals with delayed onset displayed many PTSD symptoms shortly after exposure to a traumatic event but did not exhibit a sufficient number of symptoms to exceed the diagnostic threshold.

Because traumatic stimuli have such power to evoke emotional, behavioral, and physiological reactions, it has been possible to develop treatment and research approaches in which individuals with PTSD are exposed to trauma-related stimuli in a controlled setting. Such treatments (e.g., cognitive-behavioral treatment) have proved to be very effective in ameliorating the symptoms of this disorder. In addition, laboratory research, in which subjects with PTSD are exposed to trauma-related stimuli, has furthered our understanding of the biobehavioral abnormalities associated with this disorder.

Many Japanese survivors (who had functioned well for decades) of the World War II bombing of Kobe had a relapse of PTSD symptoms following the major earthquake of 1995. They reported that the physical sensations (rumbling and tremors of the earth), the enormous death and destruction that surrounded them, and the threat to life of loved ones recalled long-dormant memories and feelings evoked by the bombing attacks 50 years earlier.

Chapter 2 *reviews specific diagnostic criteria for PTSD as well as assessment strategies and instruments.* ***Chapter 3*** *considers global treatment issues, while* ***Chapters 4 and 5*** *review psychological and pharmacological treatments (respectively) for PTSD.* ***Chapter 6*** *considers acute post-traumatic reactions, including diagnostic criteria, assessment strategies, and treatment for acute stress disorder (ASD).*

Key Concepts for Chapter 1

1. Trauma occurs not just from exposure to a catastrophic event; it also depends on the emotional response of the person exposed to such an event.

2. A person must experience trauma-related symptoms and impairments in everyday functioning for at least a month before diagnostic assessment for PTSD would be appropriate.

3. Prevalence rates for PTSD in the United States are about 6.8–7.8 percent (5 percent in men and 10 percent in women) of those exposed to catastrophic stress. Worldwide, especially where war and terrorism are common, prevalence is much higher and constitutes a major public health challenge.

4. PTSD sufferers can experience the disorder throughout their lifetime (where symptoms are chronic, severe, and permanent), occasionally (as remissions and relapses typically linked to some exposure that resembles the original trauma), and with a delayed onset (occurring months or years following exposure to a traumatic event). They may also achieve a full recovery after the initial episode and have no further problems.

Chapter 2
Recognizing, Diagnosing, and Assessing PTSD

This chapter answers the following questions:

▶ **What Are the Main Characteristics of PTSD?**

▶ **What Are the *DSM–I–TR* Diagnostic Criteria for PTSD?**—This section includes a reprint of the *DSM–IV–TR* criteria and a discussion of each major criterion.

▶ **How Should Clinicians Approach Initial Patient Interviews?**—This section covers strategies for conducting the initial clinical interview as well as PTSD risk factors to identify early in the assessment process.

▶ **What Tools Are Available for Diagnosing PTSD?**—This section presents strategies for conducting a clinical interview, identifying risk factors, and using standard measurements to assist in the PTSD diagnosis.

▶ **How Do You Differentiate PTSD from Comorbid and Other Disorders?**—This section reviews comorbid disorders and other posttraumatic outcomes as well as their prevalence. It also covers how to differentiate from PTSD both coexisting disorders and other conditions that manifest in a person who has experienced trauma.

What Are the Main Characteristics of PTSD?

As noted in Chapter 1, people at risk for PTSD have not only been exposed to a severely stressful event but have exhibited a very strong emotional reaction to this experience (characterized as fear, helplessness, or horror). Such individuals must also exhibit a pattern of symptoms embedded within three symptom "clusters"—reexperiencing, avoidance/numbing, and hyperarousal—as well as certain duration and functional impairment symptoms.

> *Figure 2.1, on page 10, provides an overview of these symptom clusters.*

Reexperiencing Symptoms

Unique to PTSD, these symptoms reflect the persistence of thoughts, feelings, and behaviors specifically related to the traumatic event. Such recollections are intrusive because they are not only unwanted but also powerful enough to negate consideration of anything else. Daytime recollections and traumatic nightmares often evoke panic, terror, dread, grief, or despair.

> *Reexperiencing can elicit symptoms of psychological distress (e.g., terror) or abnormal physiological reactions (e.g., racing pulse, rapid breathing, or sweating)*

Sometimes people with PTSD are exposed to reminders of the trauma (trauma-related stimuli) and are suddenly thrust into a psychological state—the PTSD flashback—in which they relive the traumatic experience, losing all connection with the present. This is referred to as an acute dissociative reaction, in which

Figure 2.1   PTSD Symptom Clusters

Cluster	Specific Symptoms
Reexperiencing	• Intrusive recollections • Traumatic nightmares • PTSD flashbacks • Trauma-related, stimulus-evoked psychological distress • Trauma-related, stimulus-evoked physiological reactions
Avoidance/Numbing	• Avoiding trauma-related thoughts and feelings • Avoiding trauma-related activities, places, and people • Amnesia for trauma-related memories • Diminished interest • Feeling detached or estranged • Restricted range of affect • Sense of foreshortened future
Hyperarousal	• Insomnia • Irritability • Difficulty concentrating • Hypervigilance • Exaggerated startle reaction

they actually behave as if they must fight for their lives, as was the case during exposure to the initial trauma.

For example, a woman was raped at dusk by an assailant who sprang out of the shadows opening onto an urban thoroughfare. He dragged her into the recesses of a dark alley before beginning his sexual assault. It is now many months later. She is walking home from work. The setting sun produces shadows over every nook and cranny adjacent to the sidewalk. As she glances into a heavily shadowed alley, she actually "sees" an assailant poised and ready to grab her. In fact, no one is there. The similarity between the rape scene several months ago and those produced today by an urban sunset have produced a *hallucination* that is, in effect, a PTSD flashback. As a result, she believes that she is again about to be raped and runs down the street, screaming in terror.

hallucination—a compelling perceptual experience of seeing, hearing, or smelling something that is not actually present

Avoidance/Numbing Symptoms

These symptoms can be understood as behavioral, cognitive, or emotional strategies used to ward off the terror and distress caused by reexperiencing symptoms.

Avoidance symptoms include:

▶ Efforts to avoid thoughts, feelings, activities, places, and people related to the original traumatic event

▶ *Psychogenic amnesia* for trauma-related memories (e.g., a 10-year-old refugee who witnessed the massacre of his father and brothers and the rape of his mother by armed paramilitary militia members only remembers that the troops came to the house, that he ran, hid, and eventually escaped; he cannot remember what happened in between)

Numbing symptoms are psychological mechanisms through which PTSD sufferers anesthetize themselves against the intolerable panic, terror, and pain evoked by reexperiencing symptoms. These include *psychic numbing,* in which the person suppresses all feelings in order to block out the intolerable ones. This can come at a very high price (e.g., numbing intolerable, trauma-related feelings requires also anesthetizing loving feelings necessary to sustain an intimate relationship).

Hyperarousal Symptoms

These symptoms are the most apparent manifestations of the excessive physiologic arousal that is part of the PTSD syndrome and include insomnia, irritability, *startle reactions,* and *hypervigilance.* Hyperarousal symptoms make up a *hyperreactive psychophysiological state* that makes it very difficult for people with PTSD to concentrate or perform other cognitive tasks. For example, a youth with PTSD might not be able to do schoolwork or focus on intellectual tasks. Combatants in Iraq and Afghanistan speak of "having your head on a swivel," meaning that they must be on alert (e.g., hypervigilant) at all times and must constantly survey all 360 degrees of the environment.

This cluster of PTSD symptoms most closely resembles symptoms seen in *panic disorder* and *generalized anxiety disorder* and is one reason why PTSD has been classified in *DSM–IV–TR* as an anxiety disorder. For information on distinguishing panic disorder and generalized anxiety disorder from PTSD, see pages 22–23.

What Are the *DSM–IV–TR* Diagnostic Criteria for PTSD?

To be diagnosed with PTSD, a person must have been exposed to trauma and experience symptoms for at least a month after exposure. Figure 2.2, on page 12, presents the *DSM–IV–TR* criteria for PTSD. The following provides detailed discussion and examples for these criteria.

psychogenic amnesia—the inability to remember emotionally charged events for psychological rather than neurological reasons

psychic numbing—the inability to feel any emotions, either positive (love and pleasure) or negative (fear or guilt), also described as an "emotional anesthesia"

startle reactions—"jumpy" behavior manifested as a tendency to exhibit an exaggerated startle response to unexpected noises or movements by others

hypervigilance—preoccupied by watchful or protective behavior motivated by excessive fears for personal safety

hyperreactive psychophysiological state—a state in which emotions are heightened and aroused, and even minor events may produce a state in which the heart pounds rapidly, muscles are tense, and there is great overall agitation

panic disorder—a psychiatric disorder marked by intense anxiety and panic as well as many physical symptoms such as palpitations, shortness of breath, dizziness, sweating, and a sense of impending death

generalized anxiety disorder—a psychiatric disorder marked by unrealistic worry, apprehension, and uncertainty as well as physical symptoms such as muscle tension, restlessness, dry mouth, and constant worry

Figure 2.2   *DSM–IV–TR* Diagnostic Criteria for Posttraumatic Stress Disorder[5]

A. The person has been exposed to a traumatic event in which both of the following were present:

   1. The person experienced, witnessed, or was confronted with an event or events that involved actual or threatened death or serious injury, or a threat to the physical integrity of self or others.

   2. The person's response involved intense fear, helplessness, or horror.

B. The traumatic event is persistently reexperienced in one (or more) of the following ways:

   1. Recurrent and intrusive distressing recollections of the event, including images, thoughts, or perceptions

   2. Recurrent distressing dreams of the event

   3. Acting or feeling as if the traumatic event were recurring (includes a sense of reliving the experience, illusions, hallucinations and dissociative flashback episodes) [See Chapter 1.]

   4. Intense psychological distress at exposure to internal or external cues that symbolize or resemble an aspect of the traumatic event

   5. Physiological reactivity

C. Persistent avoidance of stimuli associated with the trauma and numbing of general responsiveness (not present before the trauma), as indicated by three (or more) of the following:

   1. Efforts to avoid thoughts, feelings, or conversations associated with the trauma

   2. Efforts to avoid activities, places, or people that arouse recollections of the trauma

   3. Inability to recall an important aspect of the trauma

   4. Markedly diminished interest or participation in significant activities

   5. Feeling of detachment or estrangement from others

   6. Restricted range of affect (e.g., unable to have loving feelings)

   7. Sense of a foreshortened future (e.g., does not expect to have a career, marriage, children, or a normal life span)

D. Persistent symptoms of increased arousal not present before the trauma, as indicated by two (or more) of the following:

   1. Difficulty falling or staying asleep

   2. Irritability or outbursts of anger

   3. Difficulty concentrating

   4. Hypervigilance

   5. Exaggerated startle response

E. Duration of the disturbance (symptoms in Criteria B, C, and D) is more than 1 month.

F. The disturbance causes clinically significant distress or impairment in social, occupation, or other important areas of functioning.

  Specify:

   Acute: if duration of symptoms is less than 3 months

   Chronic: if duration of symptoms is 3 months or more

  Specify:

   With delayed onset: if onset of symptoms is at least 6 months after the stressor

Source: Reprinted with permission by the American Psychiatric Association: *Diagnostic and Statistical Manual of Mental Disorders, Fourth Edition Text Revision.* Washington, DC: American Psychiatric Association, 2000.

The Traumatic Stress Criterion

The *DSM–IV–TR* definition of a traumatic event has two components: exposure to a catastrophic event (the A_1 criterion) and emotional distress because of such exposure (the A_2 criterion).[5]

The A_1 Exposure Criterion

People who meet the *DSM–IV–TR* A_1 criterion have been exposed to catastrophic events that involve actual or threatened death or serious injury (e.g., military combat, sexual assault, physical attack, torture, man-made/natural disasters, accidents, incarceration, or exposure to war-zone/urban/domestic violence). Others meeting the A_1 criterion include people not directly endangered, but who witness such events and people who witness the violent aftermath of a catastrophic event (such as dead body parts) but were never personally in danger. Finally, *DSM–IV–TR* adds "confronted with" a life-threatening event to the A_1 criterion (e.g., someone learns that a loved one has died during a catastrophic event, but has not experienced any personal danger).

The A_2 Distress Criterion

People are different. Some people exposed to an A_1 event will experience severe psychological distress, characterized in *DSM–IV–TR* as "fear, helplessness, or horror"; others will not exhibit such distress; and still others may have a delayed response.

- ▶ **Those Who Experience Significant Distress**—Those people who exhibit intensive distress following an A_1 event meet the PTSD A_2 criterion and can be said to have been "traumatized."

- ▶ **Those Who Do Not Experience Significant Distress**—Those who cope with an A_1 event without exhibiting "fear, helplessness, or horror" do not meet the PTSD A_2 criterion, have not been "traumatized," and cannot have PTSD. This scenario often applies to people who are exposed to A_1 events continually because of their professional responsibilities (such as military, police, and emergency medical personnel), who do not meet the A_2 criterion.

A_1 events differ considerably in their capacity to evoke psychological distress; suffering injury due to willful, violent, personal intent (as in rape, assault, or torture) is much more distressing than suffering injury from an impersonal accident or natural disaster. This is a major reason why 46 percent of women who have been raped develop PTSD compared to only 9 percent of women involved in an accident.[1]

"Mothers of the Disappeared" are women whose children were arrested by police during the state-sponsored terrorism of the "Dirty War" in Argentina, when the military junta arrested, incarcerated, tortured, and often executed individuals whom they considered subversive. These mothers may or may not have witnessed any more than the arrest of their children. In all cases, however, their children's continued disappearance was a very strong indication that they might have been executed. According to DSM–IV–TR, these mothers have all suffered exposure to an A_1 event, because they have been "confronted with" the probable violent death of their children.

Children, especially those aged 6 years and younger, who lack an adult's capacity for abstract thinking or linguistic expression, may express their emotional reaction (A₂ reaction) behaviorally rather than verbally through developmentally appropriate, nonverbal indicators of psychological distress, such as disorganized or agitated behavior during play.

The case study of Mary T. (pages 15 through 17) illustrates this scenario.

Multiple Traumas

Although people may develop severe PTSD from one horrific event, as did Mary T. (see below), it is not uncommon in clinical practice to see people who have been exposed to many extremely stressful A criterion experiences. Unfortunately, this is common in cases of childhood sexual or physical trauma, domestic violence, urban violence, forced migration, war, state terrorism (e.g., as torture), or state-sponsored genocide. If the events are sequential episodes of the same traumatic stressor (as in child abuse, war, etc.), psychosocial treatment may be successful by focusing on the "worst" episode (see Chapter 4). If, however, two or more traumatic stressors are quite different in character (e.g., war trauma and childhood sexual abuse), each A criterion experience may have to be addressed separately during psychotherapy.

Although an individual need not have more than one reexperiencing (B), three avoidant/numbing (C), and two hyperarousal (D) symptoms to meet *DSM–IV–TR* diagnostic criteria for PTSD (as stated in Figure 2.3 on pages 15 through 17), it is not at all unusual for a traumatized person to exhibit most, if not all, B, C, and D symptoms.

How Should Clinicians Approach Initial Patient Interviews?

In general, PTSD is not a difficult diagnosis to make if the clinician keeps the diagnostic criteria in mind. It is essential, however, that the clinician conduct the diagnostic interview in a manner that acknowledges the patient's worst fears and that provides an environment of sensitivity, safety, and trust. After all, the clinician is asking the PTSD patient to take a tremendous risk and abandon all the avoidance behaviors and protective and other psychological strategies that buffer the patient from the intolerable memories and feelings associated with the traumatic event.

In the case of chronic PTSD, where protective layers have solidified for years or decades, the clinician must be patient and obtain the trauma history at a pace that the patient can tolerate. It is usually helpful to immediately acknowledge to the patient how difficult it must be to answer these questions. It is also helpful for the clinician to encourage the patient to indicate when the interview becomes too upsetting and to back off immediately when the patient communicates this.

Since most people who experience trauma do not develop PTSD, understanding who might be at greater risk is important. The factors listed in Figure 2.4, on page 19, are associated with greater risk for PTSD.[17,18] Although this table identifies many pretraumatic risk

Figure 2.3   Diagnosing Mary T.: A Case Study

Trauma Event Symptoms—A Criteria

Mary T. was a 27-year-old, happily married woman. One Sunday while driving to church, her car was hit by a large semi-tractor-trailer that had been unable to stop at a red light because of faulty brakes. The truck was exceeding the speed limit, its momentum was great, and the impact of the collision was tremendous. As the truck crashed into the right side of the car, her husband was killed instantly.

Mary was badly bruised but not seriously injured. Instead, she was trapped in the car for several hours before she could be extricated by the rescue squad. During that period, her dead husband was crushed against her. She was covered with his blood. It was a terrifying and horrifying experience. She recalls an overwhelming sense of loss, despair, and rage as she was trapped in the car waiting to be released but not wanting the separation from her husband that would result.

Reexperiencing Symptoms—B Criteria

After release from the emergency room and a six-week convalescence with her sister in a different city, Mary returned home determined to pick up the pieces and go on with her career as a software designer in a prestigious and very successful computer firm. In cases of PTSD, some or all of Mary's reexperiencing symptoms illustrate how the traumatic event remains, sometimes for decades, a dominating psychological experience that retains its power to evoke panic, terror, dread, grief, or despair.

Intrusive Recollections—Criterion B_1	It was extremely difficult to go to work, but she forced herself to do so, convinced that familiar surroundings, supportive colleagues, and enjoyable work would provide a much-needed distraction from the intrusive recollections exemplified by the incessant replay in her mind of the most awful moments of the accident. But she couldn't get her mind to focus on anything but images from the crash: the noise of the truck, the green traffic light, the impact of her husband's limp body, his warm, sticky blood flowing over her, and her inescapable confinement in the wrecked car.
Traumatic Nightmares—Criterion B_2	She often awoke at night in a state of panic from the same traumatic nightmare in which she was crushed by her husband's body, covered with his blood, and clawing at the shattered window trying to escape from the car.
PTSD Flashbacks—Criterion B_3	Most disturbing were the PTSD flashbacks, which generally occurred when a large truck would rumble close by, especially when she was riding in a car. At such times, she would actually "see" the truck change direction and head straight toward her. At some level, she knew that her mind was playing tricks on her and that there was no truck swerving inexorably in her direction. But during these episodes, her terror was so great and her hold on reality so weak that she could think of nothing but escape from the oncoming truck she believed would destroy her.
Intense Psychological Distress—Criterion B_4	Mary T. also found that stimuli that reminded her of the crash could produce marked psychological distress and physiological reactivity. These stimuli included driving a car, being in close proximity to large trucks, being near the intersection where the accident occurred, and being exposed to any cinematic, TV, newspaper, or fictitious depiction of a motor vehicle accident. This included TV automobile commercials depicting car crashes and automobile chase scenes in action movies. When exposed to such stimuli, she experienced intense psychological distress marked by terror, horror, overwhelming sense of loss, despair, and rage.
Physiological Reactivity—Criterion B_5	When exposed to such stimuli, she also experienced physiological reactivity marked by a pounding heart, racing pulse, rapid breathing, sweating, and an awful headache.

(continued)

Figure 2.3 (*Continued*)

Avoidance/Numbing Symptoms—C Criterion		
Thoughts and memories about the accident evoked such an intense emotional and physiological reaction that Mary made concerted efforts to avoid thoughts, feelings, or conversations about the trauma as well as activities, places, or people associated with it.		
Avoid Thoughts, Feelings, or Conversations about the Trauma—Criterion C_1		It was because she didn't want to think about the accident that Mary refused to take legal action against the trucking company that had negligently failed to inspect and repair the truck's faulty brakes. When she found herself involuntarily beginning to think about the accident, she would try to distract herself with music, work, or some other emotionally neutral matter with which she could occupy her mind.
Avoid Activities, Places, or People Associated with the Trauma—Criterion C_2		She avoided riding in a car, traveling on major roadways where she might encounter tractor-trailer trucks, and watching TV or movies for fear that they would contain crash scenes or other images reminiscent of the accident. She even tried to stay awake as long as she could at night to avoid the traumatic nightmares that terrified her three or four times each week.
Inability to Recall an Important Aspect of the Trauma—Criterion C_3		The inability to recall important aspects of the trauma (psychogenic amnesia), which may last for years, differs qualitatively from behavioral avoidance or psychic numbing. Initially, Mary was certain that she had complete recall of the entire event. After all, her problem was not amnesia, but rather that the intrusive recollections and other reexperiencing symptoms were so terribly unbearable that she couldn't work, sleep, or function as she had before the accident. However, after weeks of reviewing and reprocessing the event with her psychotherapist, she began to remember more and more details of the accident. She indeed had experienced an inability to recall an important aspect of the trauma. What she began to recall was even worse than what she had remembered. She began to have a vivid recollection of the initial impact when the nose of the truck plowed through the door, sweeping her husband into her lap. Worst still, she now recalled that he didn't die instantly but lived long enough to gaze at her imploringly, his face contorted by pain, looking at her silently, unable to speak, breathing his last, and begging for help. This was the most unbearable memory of all.
Diminished Interest and Stopped Participating—Criterion C_4		Mary T. felt that she had become a very different person since the accident, and she didn't like the changes she perceived in herself. Whereas previously she had been open, emotional, adventurous, and gregarious, she was now withdrawn, unresponsive, wooden, and solitary. She exhibited diminished interest and stopped participating in the many social, athletic, and church activities in which she had previously been very active.
Detached and Estranged From Others—Criterion C_5		She felt detached and estranged from others, especially from her sister and two closest friends, partially because she was convinced that no one could possibly know or understand how her old self had been irreversibly changed by the accident. It was, therefore, impossible for her to maintain interpersonal relationships as before. She didn't want to be with others and actively resisted their efforts to spend time with her.
Restricted Range of Affect—Criterion C_6		She felt numb, wooden, and hollow inside, as if her capacity for emotional experience and expression had been completely anesthetized. This restricted range of affect made it impossible for Mary to enjoy companionship or reciprocate feelings of warmth, friendship, intimacy, or love.
Fore-shortened Future—Criterion C_7		Finally, she felt that her life was over, that she had a foreshortened future with no career, marriage, children, or normal life span to look forward to.

Figure 2.3 (*Continued*))

Hyperarousal Symptoms—D Criterion		
Mary T. was in a state of constant arousal, agitation, and anxiety. Others perceived her as being jumpy, nervous, easily upset, and having a hair-trigger temper. She had difficulty falling or staying asleep.		
Difficulty Falling or Staying Asleep— Criterion D_1	Insomnia occurred either because she couldn't distract her mind from intrusive recollections of the trauma, because she was awakened by traumatic nightmares, or because her high level of physiological overdrive was too much to permit sleep.	
Irritability or Outbursts of Anger— Criterion D_2	She exhibited irritability or outbursts of anger that astonished friends who had previously regarded her as an easy-going and resilient individual with a great sense of humor.	
Difficulty Concentrating— Criterion D_3	She had difficulty concentrating because her mind was preoccupied with intrusive recollections or because her arousal level was so high that she could not focus on any intellectual task for a sustained period. This was such a problem that she had to take a leave of absence from her job.	
Hypervigilance— Criterion D_4	Mary became obsessed with fears about personal safety. The tragic and traumatic accident that had killed her husband made her hypervigilant for the first sign of danger. This was especially noticeable when she was in a car, but it also included being reluctant to go shopping alone, refusing to venture out of her house after dark, and installing an elaborate security system in her home.	
An Exaggerated Startle Response— Criterion D_5	Finally, she was extremely jumpy and would exhibit an exaggerated startle response to any unexpected noise. The exquisitely sensitive startle reflex is a well-understood adaptive response to trauma that has been studied extensively in both animal and human research.	
Clinically Significant Distress and Impairment—F Criterion		
Mary T.'s PTSD caused clinically significant distress and impairment socially (e.g., withdrawal from friends, relationships, and activities), occupationally (e.g., a leave of absence from work because of her inability to function), and in other important areas of functioning. Therefore, she met the functional impairment (F) criterion.		
Diagnosis: Chronic PTSD		
Mary T. has chronic PTSD because her symptoms persisted much longer than three months.		

personality pathology—maladaptive pattern of relating to other people that severely impairs social functioning and adaptive potential

peritraumatic dissociation—dissociation during and shortly after the trauma

psychometric instruments—tests that measure psychological factors, such as personality, intelligence, beliefs, and fears

factors, they have only modest power as PTSD predictors. Research indicates that the strongest risk factors were severity ("dose") of the trauma and poor posttraumatic social support.[17]

What Tools Are Available for Diagnosing PTSD?

Assessing the possible presence of PTSD may require several meetings in which the clinician conducts a careful diagnostic interview, asks questions about risk factors for PTSD, and rules out other possible disorders. Well-validated screening instruments are available for identifying individuals at risk for PTSD, especially in primary care settings (see Appendix: Table 1). A positive screen should never be considered a positive diagnosis. It simply identifies those individuals who should receive a more definitive evaluation. Additionally, clinicians may utilize assessment tools, such as structured interviews or *psychometric instruments*. Instruments for assessing exposure to trauma, for diagnosing, and for determining the severity of PTSD symptoms in adults and children are often utilized and may improve diagnostic accuracy.

Using Structured Interviews and Questionnaires

Many structured interviews and questionnaires exist for assessing and diagnosing PTSD. Comprehensive tables that list recommended screening and assessment instruments for adults and children (and adolescents) can be found in the Appendix. These instruments fall into three overlapping categories:

1. **Trauma Exposure Scales** determine exposure to a criterion A_1 event by documenting the nature and severity of such overwhelming stressors. General exposure questionnaires inquire about exposure to all possible kinds of catastrophic events, while specific exposure

From the Patient's Perspective

Well, I did it! I sat through two hours with that psychologist. I couldn't believe there were so many questions. I also couldn't believe that so many of them seemed to fit. Right on target about all that's been bothering me. I did pretty well at first. And I didn't mind telling her what a mess I've been. How my nerves are shot. The nightmares. And all the rest. But when she started asking about the accident, I lost it. I just couldn't go on. And I'm getting so upset just thinking about it that I'd better stop right now.

Figure 2.4   Risk Factors for PTSD

<table>
<tr>
<td rowspan="8">Pretraumatic</td>
<td>

- **Gender**—Women are twice as likely as men to develop PTSD at some point in their lives, partially due to the likelihood of experiencing interpersonal violence (e.g., rape, sexual molestation, parental neglect, childhood sexual/physical abuse). That doesn't appear to be the case among American female military personnel in Iraq and Afghanistan where PTSD prevalence is no greater than with males.
- **Age**—Adults younger than 25 are most at risk.
- **Education**—Those with less than a college education are more at risk.
- **Childhood Trauma**—Child abuse (including sexual abuse), rape, war, or motor vehicle accidents can increase risk.
- **Childhood Adversity**—Economic deprivation or parental separation/divorce before the child is age 10 **years** can be a factor.
- **Adverse Life Events**—Divorce, loss of job, failure at school, financial problems, or poor physical health can increase risk.
- **Psychiatric Disorders**—Those diagnosed with a childhood conduct disorder (e.g., attention deficit hyperactivity disorder) or those with any prior psychiatric disorder are most at risk, as are those with a *personality pathology*.
- **Genetics**—Family history of any psychiatric disorder or possible genetic differences in regulating presynaptic uptake of serotonin (or other neurobiological mechanisms) can increase risk.*

</td>
</tr>
<tr>
<td rowspan="5">Traumatic</td>
<td>

- **Severity ("Dose") of the Trauma**—The greater the magnitude of trauma exposure, the greater the likelihood of developing PTSD.
- **Nature of the Trauma**—Interpersonal violence (e.g., rape, physical attack, torture, war-zone trauma) in which there is a human perpetrator is much more likely to produce PTSD than an impersonal event (e.g., natural disaster).
- **Betrayal**—When a parent or caregiver on whom the victim is completely dependent perpetrates interpersonal violence, as in childhood sexual abuse, the trauma is more likely to produce PTSD than when the perpetrator is a stranger.
- *Peritraumatic Dissociation*—This symptom, as seen in acute stress disorder (ASD), is more likely to predict the later development of PTSD than if the trauma survivor did not experience dissociative symptoms at the time of the trauma.
- **Participation in Atrocities**—Being either a perpetrator or witness of atrocities has proven to be a risk factor for Vietnam and other military veterans.

</td>
</tr>
<tr>
<td rowspan="3">Posttraumatic</td>
<td>

- **Poor Social Support**—After exposure to trauma, lack of social support is a risk factor for the onset of PTSD.
- **Development of Acute Stress Disorder (ASD)**—ASD is a strong indication of posttraumatic symptom severity and predicts the later development of PTSD among 80 percent of affected individuals (see Chapter 6).
- **Access to Acute, Posttraumatic Clinical Intervention**—As discussed in Chapter 6, timely treatment of ASD can prevent the later development of PTSD.

</td>
</tr>
</table>

* Genetic research has shown that, of the two variants of the gene regulating presynaptic uptake of serotonin, the long form appears to be associated with resilience and the short form with vulnerability to stressful events. Individuals who inherited the short form and were exposed to four or more stressful life events were much more likely to develop PTSD or depression or to attempt suicide.[20] Other genes that may confer vulnerability or resilience are currently under investigation. Studies of twins have also indicated that there is a genetic vulnerability to PTSD.[21]

scales may focus on child abuse, domestic violence, rape, combat exposure, or torture. (See Appendix: Table 2 for adults and Table 5 for children and adolescents.)

2. **Diagnostic Instruments** take the form of structured interviews administered by a clinician or lay interviews designed for survey research. These often broad-spectrum instruments inquire about all *DSM–IV–TR* diagnoses with a separate specific module dedicated to PTSD diagnostic criteria. Such instruments may also detect comorbid diagnoses. (See Appendix: Table 3 for adults and Table 6 for children and adolescents.)

3. **Symptom Severity Scales** are primarily available for PTSD, usually as self-report questionnaires in which individuals indicate (usually on a four- or five-point scale) the intensity of a specific PTSD symptom (such as traumatic nightmares). (See Appendix: Table 4 for adults and Table 7 for children and adolescents.)

In practice, it is usually best to start with a general trauma exposure scale. If the patient reports previous exposure to a criterion A_1 event, one can either inquire in more detail about the specific trauma exposure (e.g., child abuse) or proceed directly to a diagnostic instrument to determine whether PTSD is present. PTSD severity can next be determined with a symptom severity scale or with the Clinician Administered PTSD Scale (CAPS), which is both a diagnostic instrument and symptom severity scale.

Within this class of instruments are structured clinical interviews that can be used both as diagnostic instruments and symptom severity scales (e.g., the Clinician Administered PTSD Scale [CAPS]).

A thorough and comprehensive discussion of PTSD assessment can be found in an excellent book devoted entirely to this topic as well as in a recent comprehensive review.[22]

How Do You Differentiate PTSD from Comorbid and Other Disorders?

A victim of trauma may suffer from *comorbid* psychiatric disorders in addition to PTSD, or the trauma may result in a disorder that is different from PTSD.

comorbid disorders—major psychiatric disorders that are present at the same time as full-fledged PTSD

Other Axis I Psychiatric Syndromes—Individuals with lifetime PTSD likely meet *DSM–IV–TR* diagnostic criteria for at least one other Axis I psychiatric disorder. Indeed, 80 percent of all men and women with lifetime PTSD in the National Comorbidity Study also met criteria for at least one of the following: major depressive disorder, dysthymia, generalized anxiety disorder, simple phobia, social phobia, panic disorder, alcohol abuse/dependence, drug abuse/dependence, or conduct disorder.[1]

Comorbidity is important to keep in mind when conducting a diagnostic assessment or formulating a treatment plan for someone suspected of having PTSD.

Figure 2.5, on page 21, illustrates prevalence rates for comorbid disorders. One reason for such high prevalence of comorbid disorders is the symptom overlap between PTSD and these other Axis I diagnoses.

Figure 2.5 *DSM–IV–TR* **Disorders Frequently Comorbid with PTSD**

Diagnosis	Lifetime Prevalence (%)
Major Depressive Disorder	48
Dysthymia	22
Generalized Anxiety Disorder	16
Simple Phobia	30
Social Phobia	28
Panic Disorder	12.6 vs. 7.3*
Agoraphobia	22.4 vs. 16.1*
Alcohol Abuse/Dependence	51.9 vs. 27.9**
Drug Abuse/Dependence	34.5 vs. 26.9**
Conduct Disorder	43.3 vs. 15.4**

*women > men
**men > women
Source: From the *National Comorbidity Survey.*

Traumatic Brain Injury

Recent military service in Iraq and Afghanistan has occasioned a new complication in diagnosing (and treating) PTSD among men and women who have sustained concussive injuries from roadside bombs, suicide bombers, or proximity to other explosions. Indeed, any attack intense enough to produce traumatic brain injury (TBI) has the psychological potential to produce PTSD due to life threat and witnessing the death or injury of others. For this reason, clinicians in military settings and VA hospitals are often challenged by patients who simultaneously exhibit the symptoms of both PTSD and TBI. It should be understood that a history of TBI indicates the severity of the concussive injury at the time it occurred; it provides no information about the current status of the individual regarding the presence or severity of post-concussive symptoms. As most people exposed to psychological trauma do not develop PTSD, most people who experience TBI do not develop persistent post-concussive symptoms

The vast majority of concussive injuries meet the criteria for mild (as distinguished from moderate and severe) TBI. Mild TBI may be especially difficult to distinguish from PTSD since both conditions are often marked by problems with concentration, memory, irritability, insomnia, and other behavioral changes. Furthermore, the memory, concentration and headache problems ordinarily seen in mild TBI are seen much more frequently if the TBI is associated with PTSD. This is an urgent clinical challenge that has stimulated a great deal of research to determine both optimal assessment strategies, as well as effective treatment approaches.[23]

Other Posttraumatic Problems

There is growing evidence that PTSD may not be the only clinically significant consequence of exposure to a catastrophic event. Other types of posttraumatic outcomes discussed should also receive clinician/researcher attention. Furthermore, some people exposed to traumatic stress never exhibit PTSD. Instead, they may develop depression, alcoholism, or some other *DSM–IV–TR* disorder.

> **Medical Disorders**—Growing evidence indicates that exposure to catastrophic events is a risk factor for many medical disorders affecting the cardiovascular, gastrointestinal, endocrinological, musculoskeletal, and other bodily systems.[12,24]

> **Partial/Subsyndromal PTSD**—There is growing interest in people who lack only one or two of the three mandatory *DSM–IV–TR* symptoms. A number of studies have shown that such individuals have clinically significant, posttraumatic symptoms and functional impairment even though they do not meet diagnostic criteria for PTSD.[25–27]

> **Complex PTSD**—Prolonged trauma, especially childhood sexual abuse or torture during political incarceration, may produce a clinical syndrome that differs considerably from that seen in PTSD. This syndrome, provisionally called "complex PTSD," features impulsivity, dissociation, *somatization*, *affect lability*, interpersonal difficulties, and *pathological changes* in personal identity (dissociative identity disorder in *DSM–IV*; previously multiple personality disorder in *DSM–III*).[28]

There is growing evidence that PTSD may not be the only clinically significant consequence of exposure to a catastrophic event. Differentiating PTSD symptoms from other disorders involves considering factors such as the following:

1. **Affective Disorders**—PTSD patients may exhibit symptoms similar to depression or dysthymia (insomnia, impaired concentration, social withdrawal, and diminished interest in activities). However, affective disorders are characterized more by depressed mood, decreased capacity for enjoyment, guilt, weight loss, suicidal thoughts, and a slowing of thoughts and actions (e.g., "psychomotor retardation").

2. **Generalized Anxiety Disorder (GAD)**—Patients with PTSD exhibit irritability, hypervigilance, exaggerated startle response, impaired concentration, insomnia, and autonomic hyperarousal; however, GAD is more likely if there is the presence of unrealistic worry, muscle ten-

somatization—the expression of emotional distress through physical symptoms such as peptic ulcer, asthma, or chronic pain

affect lability—rapid and unpredictable shifts in mood state

pathological changes—changes resulting in an abnormal condition that prevents proper psychological functioning

sion, restlessness, dry mouth, frequent urination, and a lump in the throat.

3. **Phobias** (e.g., simple phobia, social phobia, and agoraphobia)—Although some patients exhibit both avoidant and arousal behaviors typical of PTSD, perhaps triggered by environmental and/or social stimuli, phobia patients do not exhibit the numbing symptoms seen in PTSD.

4. **Panic Disorder**—Symptoms of panic disorder resemble those of PTSD because they include many symptoms of autonomic hyperarousal and because panic patients may exhibit dissociation. In contrast to stimulus-driven PTSD symptoms, however, panic attacks are unexpected and occur spontaneously; they are associated with symptoms of choking, numbness, tingling, fear of going crazy, and fear of dying.

5. **Chemical Abuse/Dependency**—Often seen in PTSD patients as a comorbid diagnosis, there are no symptoms concerning use and misuse of alcohol or drugs that are part of the PTSD diagnostic criteria.

Phobia patients become aroused only when they believe they will be exposed to the feared stimulus or situation. PTSD patients, on the other hand, are perpetually in a state of hyperarousal.

Key Concepts for Chapter 2

1. *DSM–IV–TR* criteria for PTSD require that, for at least a month after being exposed to a traumatic event, a person suffers intense emotional responses, persistently reexperiences elements of the event, regularly avoids stimuli associated with the trauma, becomes somewhat "numb," and suffers increased arousal.

2. PTSD symptoms must cause significant distress or impairment in social, occupational, or other important areas of functioning.

3. Diagnosis and assessment must be conducted in an environment of sensitivity, safety, and trust for the patient to be able to recount information about the traumatic event and its aftermath.

4. Those who may be more likely to develop PTSD following exposure to a traumatic event are women, young adults, those with a personal or family history of psychiatric disorders, and people who have experienced childhood trauma/adversity or adverse life events as adults.

5. The severity and nature of the trauma can significantly impact one's risk of developing PTSD.

6. Onset of PTSD following exposure to a traumatic event is more likely if the person has developed (and especially has not been treated for) acute stress disorder as well as if the person lacks social support.

7. There are a variety of tools available for assessing and diagnosing PTSD, including trauma exposure scales, diagnostic instruments, and symptom severity scales.

8. Mental health disorders typically comorbid with PTSD are major depressive disorder, dysthymia, other anxiety disorders, substance abuse, and conduct disorder. Additionally, PTSD sufferers tend to experience a variety of medical disorders.

9. Military personnel recently deployed to Iraq and Afghanistan may sustain traumatic brain injuries, which may or may not occur simultaneously with PTSD. This is a very important challenge for diagnosis and treatment.

Chapter 3
Global Treatment Issues for PTSD

This chapter answers the following questions:

▶ **What Are the Timing and Priority Issues Related to Treatment?**—This section covers issues surrounding the timing of when patients seek treatment as well as priorities in PTSD treatment (e.g., psychiatric emergency, alcohol or drug abuse/dependence, comorbidity, and situational factors).

▶ **What General Considerations Exist for Choosing a Specific Treatment Option?**—This section provides an overview of treatment considerations, such as combining treatments, comorbid disorders, and complex PTSD.

▶ **What PTSD Treatment-Focus Issues Exist?**—This section covers decision making on trauma vs. supportive therapy, using combined treatments, and other issues.

▶ **What Are the Major Personal Issues for Clinicians Treating Those with PTSD?**—This section discusses therapeutic neutrality, advocacy, secondary traumatization, countertransference, and clinician self-care.

AFTER determining that a patient requesting treatment has PTSD, there are a number of questions clinicians need to address. In most respects, these questions are no different from those about other psychiatric disorders, although the presence of PTSD sometimes raises questions about treatment timing priorities, focus, and approach.

What Are the Timing and Priority Issues Related to Treatment?

For clinicians, global treatment issues often begin with answering the question, "Why seek help now?" and proceed to determining what issues or situations may delay or alter a typical PTSD treatment approach.

Timing Issues for Seeking Treatment

When people complain about the recent onset of reexperiencing, avoidant/numbing, or hyperarousal symptoms, it is usually pretty obvious why they are seeking treatment at this time and that PTSD is the first (and possibly only) order of business. On the other hand, when people who have had chronic PTSD for many years suddenly request treatment, it is usually because something has changed abruptly in their lives. This change has disrupted their equilibrium in terms of coping both with PTSD symptoms and the demands of family, friends, work, and society.

Sometimes the precipitant is obvious; however, at other times, the clinician must take a careful history to identify the recent precipitant. For example:

▶ A Red Cross disaster worker complains of traumatic nightmares related to an event she or he had not thought about for a long time. It is likely that certain specific details of a recent disaster reactivated memories of a similar event in the past, about which there remain intense, unresolved emotional feelings.

▶ A woman who has successfully dealt with the emotional consequences of her own childhood sexual abuse begins having intrusive recollections of this traumatic experience when her adolescent daughter begins dating or becomes sexually active.

▶ A military veteran may experience a reexacerbation of symptoms when television coverage focuses on new military offensives (e.g., Iraq, Afghanistan) or when his or her child is called up for military duty.

▶ For older veterans, the death of an adult child (even by natural causes such as cancer) may reactivate survival guilt about having outlived friends at Normandy Beach or in Vietnam.

Some trauma-related stimuli can be heavily disguised. Take the example of a successful businesswoman with a *well-encapsulated* sexual trauma history that has caused no previous emotional difficulty. She may suddenly develop PTSD symptoms when her professional advancement seems unfairly and consistently blocked by hostile or oppressive male superiors, leaving her feeling powerless. Although the precipitating stressor is in the workplace, her nightmares are inexplicably (to her) about the sexual abuse she suffered decades earlier.

well encapsulated—
psychological buffers that prevent a person from experiencing current distress from a previous traumatic event

From the Patient's Perspective

I've got to hand it to her. She asked about everything. About how depressed I've been. About how hard this has been on my relationships. And about possible problems that never would have occurred to me, like drinking and such. But at the end, she decided, and I agreed, that the major problem was the PTSD and that we really needed to consider how this accident has turned my life upside down.

Priority Issues for Treatment

In the preceding examples, PTSD is clearly the first order of business, and the clinician must develop a treatment plan that addresses both the current precipitant as well as unresolved past traumatic issues that have become central to the current clinical problem. Sometimes, however, PTSD may not be the first order of business because other clinical issues must take priority before PTSD treatment can be initiated. Common reasons for delaying PTSD treatment include the existence of:

> ► A psychiatric emergency (the patient is suicidal, homicidal, or otherwise so out of control that he or she needs the safety, structure, and control of an inpatient hospital setting)
>
> ► Serious alcohol or drug abuse/dependence or comorbid disorder that must be treated before PTSD
>
> ► A marital/familial/workplace crisis that demands immediate attention

In a psychiatric emergency, where the patient must be hospitalized without delay, a discharge plan can be developed that will implement PTSD treatment along with other necessary measures when the patient is ready to leave the hospital.

What General Considerations Exist for Choosing a Specific Treatment Option?

When creating a treatment plan for someone with PTSD, there are a number of factors to consider, including the following:

> ► **Combined Treatment**—To provide the best possible care for patients, clinicians often combine different therapies (e.g., individual therapy and medication).
>
> ► **Treatment of Comorbid Disorders**—Treatments may need to be chosen that address multiple disorders at the same time.
>
> ► **Treating "Complex PTSD"**—For those who experienced severe trauma, an alternative clinical syndrome has been proposed, perhaps demanding a longer-term treatment plan.[28–29]
>
> ► **Cross-Cultural Considerations**—Clinicians need to be sensitive to cultural differences in PTSD assessment and treatment.
>
> ► **Recovered Memories**—Controversy exists over whether previously forgotten traumatic memories can be recovered many years later as well as how such memories should be addressed by clinicians.
>
> ► **Safety**—PTSD patients often feel that it is dangerous for them to relinquish the cognitive, emotional, and behavioral avoidance strategies they habitually use to distance

Clinicians must establish an atmosphere of trust and safety, thereby "earning the right to gain access" to carefully guarded traumatic material.[31]

themselves from intolerable intrusive recollections and arousal symptoms.

What PTSD Treatment-Focus Issues Exist?

Many treatments for PTSD encourage the patient to specifically remember and focus on the experienced trauma (trauma focus treatment). Others encourage the patient to increase coping skills for current here-and-now stressors to improve daily functioning and decrease PTSD symptoms (supportive therapy). Sometimes, therapy is combined with medication. And sometimes, comorbid disorders must be treated before PTSD treatment can begin.

Trauma Focus

Trauma focus therapy uses the in-depth exploration of traumatic material to facilitate healing. As described in Chapter 4, pages 32 through 38, it can be conducted in individual or group contexts with techniques that vary from *cognitive-behavioral therapy*[30] (CBT) to *psychodynamic approaches*.[31–32] The goal of trauma focus therapy is for patients to take control of their lives by gaining authority over traumatic memories.

Trauma Focus vs. Supportive Therapy

Trauma focus treatment may not be beneficial for everyone. Most research data on trauma focus treatments apply only to those patients who have agreed to undergo such treatment. Scientific evidence shows that trauma-focused treatments (such as prolonged exposure [PE] and cognitive processing therapy [CPT]) have proven to be the most effective treatments to date. Eye-movement desensitization and reprocessing (EMDR) is another trauma focus approach in which the patient does not have to verbally recount the traumatic experience while focusing on such memories (see Chapter 4). Despite the proven efficacy of these approaches, some patients have absolutely no wish to revisit traumatic material because they:

- ▶ Want to put the past behind them
- ▶ Fear that they cannot tolerate the intrusive and arousal symptoms exacerbated by such memories

Stress inoculation training (SIT) is an alternative that has not been tested extensively. It is an evidence-based treatment that compares favorably with effective trauma focus approaches but that does not require the patient to recall painful traumatic memories. Instead, SIT emphasizes anxiety management skills to en-

cognitive-behavioral approaches—therapeutic approaches that focus on patterns of reinforcement, learning and conditioning models, and correcting erroneous cognitions

psychodynamic approaches—therapeutic approaches that focus on unconscious and conscious motivations and drives

For more information on CBT and other treatment approaches, see Chapter 4, pages 32 through 38.

able patients to cope more effectively with current situations that are predictably exacerbated by their PTSD symptoms.

Most non-focus PTSD treatments are less rigorous than SIT. What they have in common is that they encourage skill building and problem solving for current issues in the patient's life as an avenue for increasing adaptive functioning and regaining a sense of control. Supportive treatments that deliberately avoid traumatic material may be beneficial for some with PTSD, although their efficacy has yet to be demonstrated. Currently, there are no guidelines for determining which patients will most likely benefit from one kind of therapy over the other.

The superiority of trauma focus treatments, especially PE and CPT, has been endorsed by all comprehensive clinical practice guidelines for PTSD treatment that have been developed by the International Society for Traumatic Stress Studies, the American Psychiatric Association, the UK's National Institute for Clinical Excellence (NICE), Australia's Centre for Mental Health, the U.S. Institute of Medicine, and jointly by the U.S. Department of Defense and Veterans Affairs.[33–38]

These treatments are the following:

- ▶ **Psychoeducational approaches,** in which patients learn about common symptoms and experiences suffered by those with PTSD
- ▶ **Individual psychotherapies,** which focus on PTSD symptoms through various methods, such as cognitive-behavioral therapy (CBT), eye-movement desensitization reprocessing (EMDR), or psychodynamic psychotherapy
- ▶ **Group therapies,** in which trauma survivors learn about PTSD and help each other with the aid of a professional clinician
- ▶ **Treatments for children** that are age-appropriate interventions, often extrapolated from adult treatment methods
- ▶ **Other treatments** that have not been systematically tested with PTSD patients, such as couples/family therapy, hypnosis, and social rehabilitative therapies

Combined Treatment

Clinicians often combine treatment methods. For example, medication combined with individual psychotherapy treatment may not only ameliorate psychobiological abnormalities associated with PTSD, but also sufficiently reduce symptoms so patients can participate in trauma focus treatment. Some patients receive individual treatment plus marital, family, or group therapy, while others may take medication as well.

An important question is whether patients can benefit from trauma focus treatment when their lives remain dangerous because of military deployment, dangerous occupations, physical/sexual abuse, domestic violence, or otherwise unsafe living situations. Traditionally, trauma focus treatment is not provided to such patients until their lives become safer. Instead, supportive therapy and medication treatment (see Chapter 5) are generally considered better immediate options, and trauma focus therapy is delayed until personal safety can be attained. This practice is currently being reconsidered, especially by military leaders who would like to know whether troops with PTSD can benefit from trauma focus treatment while remaining in the war zone.

Chapter 4 presents detailed information on psychological treatment approaches for PTSD.

Unfortunately, there are very few published studies in which combined therapy is compared with either psychotherapy or pharmacotherapy alone. One study indicates that, among medication partial responders, outcomes improve significantly when prolonged exposure is combined with medication.[39] Another study suggests that the effectiveness of PE could be enhanced if it were combined with the medication d-cycloserine (see Chapter 5).[40]

When considering combined treatment, however, it is important to be selective and to recognize that many patients do not need more than one form of treatment at any one time.[41] Good clinical practice requires introducing only one therapeutic approach at a time and carefully gauging its effectiveness before combining it with another.

Treatment of Comorbid Disorders

Most patients with PTSD will have at least one comorbid psychiatric disorder; therefore, the treatment approach should seek to ameliorate both PTSD and the comorbid disorder(s), if possible.

Alcohol or Drug Abuse/Dependence

It is a waste of time to initiate PTSD treatment when someone is too caught up in the addiction intoxication/withdrawal cycle to participate meaningfully in any psychotherapeutic initiative. Many clinicians refuse to work with patients if they come to appointments intoxicated or if they are unable to work in psychotherapy because of their alcohol or drug abuse/dependency. If the chemical abuse/dependency is severely disruptive, patients may need to undergo inpatient detoxification and post-detoxification alcohol or drug rehabilitation (which often includes a commitment to attend Alcoholics Anonymous or Narcotics Anonymous meetings).

Clinicians must prepare and protect their patients from the fantasy that once sobriety has been achieved, all will be well. Sadly, the opposite is sometimes the case for patients with PTSD. This is because alcohol and (prescription or illicit) drug abuse often serve to blunt or numb intolerable PTSD reexperiencing or hyperarousal symptoms. During the acute withdrawal period within the first few days of detoxification, previous alcohol/drug-suppressed PTSD symptoms come raging to the forefront of conscious awareness.[42] More importantly, the PTSD patient who has successfully undergone detoxification is now suddenly thrust into the world without this protection. This is why simultaneous treatment is so important.

At the present time, it is recommended that patients with comorbid PTSD and substance use disorder (SUD) receive PE or CPT if they are neither too physically dependent nor too intoxi-

---

Pharmacotherapy, in which patients receive medications to help manage PTSD symptoms, is covered in detail in Chapter 5.

It appears that treatments that address comorbid alcohol/drug abuse/dependence and PTSD simultaneously are preferable to addressing each problem separately. Unfortunately, simultaneous treatments are generally untested, not widely available, and challenging, as each disorder exacerbates the other.[42]

cated to participate in the treatment protocol. Seeking Safety is a treatment developed specifically for people with PTSD/SUD comorbidity. Although it is popular with therapists and patients as a good first-stage treatment, its efficacy for either PTSD or SUD has yet to be established.[43]

Coexisting Psychiatric Disorders

Eighty percent of people who ever suffer from PTSD have at least one other psychiatric disorder during their lives. As a result, clinicians must consider whether to treat comorbid disorders before or along with PTSD. Sometimes the severity of the comorbid disorder demands initial attention. For example, a severely depressed individual (with comorbid PTSD) may need aggressive depression treatment, such as medication, before PTSD treatment can be considered. The same holds true for people with an immobilizing panic disorder, individuals whose eating disorder has seriously compromised their health, or persons with other psychiatric problems that are currently more incapacitating or potentially dangerous than the PTSD.

Similarly, some family, vocational, or environmental situations may require intervention before addressing PTSD. For example:

▶ A woman whose PTSD is the result of ongoing domestic violence is a poor candidate for psychotherapy, especially CBT, as long as she remains in an abusive relationship. Here, the first order of business is providing a safe and secure living situation (e.g., a battered women's shelter or safe house).

▶ A marriage on the brink of collapse because of one member's PTSD symptoms needs couples therapy before starting individual therapy for the PTSD sufferer.

▶ An employee who was injured at work and is still asked to work in conditions perceived to be unsafe has PTSD symptoms continually stirred up by such workplace conditions. The immediate challenge is to reduce incapacitating anxiety before PTSD treatment can begin. This could be accomplished by reassignment to another work site, by changes in the working environment, or by a medical/psychiatric leave of absence.

Military personnel in a war zone who do not make a timely recovery from acute stress reactions (see Chapter 6) may need to be removed to the safety of a rear echelon medical unit where they can receive appropriate intervention.

Environmental Considerations

PTSD does not occur in a vacuum. People with PTSD live in families as husbands, wives, parents, and children. They occupy positions in the workplace as employers or employees. They are often students and sometimes faculty members at schools and training facilities. It is very likely that their PTSD symptoms will have a significant effect on their family, vocational, and scholastic functioning.

Because the greatest exposure to others usually occurs in a family context, it is here that the impact of PTSD may be greatest. Individuals with PTSD are often unable to experience loving feelings or reciprocate those of partners, children, or parents. They avoid interpersonal contact. As a result, they isolate themselves and become emotionally inaccessible to those to whom they had previously been very close. They may also alienate partners and children (especially adolescents) through over-controlling and overprotective behaviors, which are a manifestation of their hypervigilance. They also cut themselves off from friends. This is especially unfortunate since social support is one of the strongest protective factors against the development of maintenance of PTSD. Furthermore development of effective marital or family therapy for PTSD is at a very preliminary stage (see Chapter 4).

At work or at school, people with PTSD may not be able to function effectively because of inability to concentrate, irritability, loss of interest in work or school, or lack of sleep. There are current efforts to ease the transition back to civilian life for active duty and military reservists who have seen recent action in Iraq and Afghanistan by working with employers on the one hand and school officials on the other. The hope is that through these efforts employers, teachers, and institutional administrators will know what problems might emerge among newly returned employees and students. Ideally, there will be employee assistance programs or campus organizations poised and ready to provide needed assistance when indicated. It is gratifying that there is such an unprecedented level of concern in the workplace and in school settings but, at present, these efforts are preliminary, at best.

Finally, there are current efforts directed at elementary school teachers who may have children of deployed or previously deployed men and women in their classrooms. Here the hope is that if a previously top student is now getting failing grades or if a previously well-behaved pupil has become a classroom nuisance or if a child is suddenly making frequent visits to the nurse's office for a variety of vague complaints, that school nurses and guidance counselors will determine, as part of their initial assessment, whether the dramatic change in behavior might be related to parental military activity. If so, it should suggest a very different approach than might be the usual response for such problems.

"Complex PTSD"

Many clinicians who work with victims of prolonged trauma, such as incest and torture, argue that these patients suffer from a clinical syndrome named "Complex PTSD" (see Chapter 2), which is not adequately characterized by the current PTSD construct.[28] The non-PTSD symptoms that comprise complex PTSD include:

▶ **Behavioral difficulties** (e.g., impulsivity, aggression, sexual acting out, eating disorders, alcohol/drug abuse, and self-destructive actions)

▶ **Emotional difficulties** (e.g., affective lability, rage, depression, and panic)

▶ **Cognitive difficulties** (e.g., *fragmented thoughts*, dissociation, and *amnesia*)

▶ **Somatization** (e.g., physical symptoms and pain)

▶ **Identity confusion** (previously called multiple personalities)

The validity of complex PTSD as a unique diagnostic entity is controversial. Many PTSD experts point out that there is very little scientific support for this diagnosis and that the vast majority of patients with complex PTSD have already met diagnostic criteria for PTSD. They also often meet diagnostic criteria for borderline personality disorder, somatization disorder, and dissociative identity disorder.[28] Complex PTSD was not included in the *DSM–IV* because it was judged that there was insufficient evidence to support its validity and utility as a unique diagnostic entity.

Proponents of the complex PTSD construct suggest that treatment for complex PTSD usually requires long-term individual and group therapies focusing on family function, vocational rehabilitation, social skills training, and alcohol/drug rehabilitation.[28] Dialectical behavior therapy (see page 40) has also been proposed as an effective treatment for complex PTSD.[44]

Cross-Cultural Considerations

PTSD has been criticized from a cross-cultural perspective as a Euro-American construct that fails to take into account culture-specific causes of stress that might be seen in trauma survivors from more traditional cultures. Some symptoms fall outside strict *DSM–IV–TR* diagnostic criteria (such as dissociative and somatic symptoms) but appear to be dramatic indications of clinically significant posttraumatic distress in their own right.[45–48] For example, in Latin America, people are diagnosed with *calor* and *ataques de nervios*.

Clinicians need to be attuned to such culture-specific idioms of distress so that they can identify posttraumatic distress when appropriate. It is also essential that, having made the diagnosis, clinicians initiate a culturally sensitive variant of PTSD treatment that will work. For example, an egalitarian approach to family

fragmented thoughts—the inability to sustain continuity and coherence in one's cognitive processes

amnesia—mental syndrome characterized by partial or complete memory loss

calor—a stress-related syndrome observed among Salvadoran women described as a surge of intense heat that may rapidly spread throughout the entire body for a few moments or for several days

ataques de nervios—a common symptom of distress among Hispanic American groups involving anxiety, uncontrollable shouting and crying, trembling, heart palpitations, difficulty breathing, dizziness, fainting spells, and dissociative symptoms (e.g., amnesia and alteration of consciousness)

Several resources offer detailed discussions of culturally sensitive treatment for trauma survivors.[45–48]

therapy is incomprehensible in some cultures where the father holds a position of authority that cannot be challenged. Likewise, clinicians pressuring for overt discussion of sexual trauma by unmarried Islamic women in group therapy fail to recognize the shameful and potentially socially disastrous consequences of such disclosure.

Recovered Memories

Controversy exists as to whether a person can recover trauma memories, that had been forgotten, many years after the trauma occurred.[49] Adults who had been sexually assaulted as children sometimes have no memories of these childhood assaults.[43] Sometimes, such missing traumatic memories later become accessible so that patients then recall traumatic childhood events such as father-daughter incest.[49–51]

A balanced review of recovered memories can be found in Posttraumatic Stress Disorder: Malady or Myth? *by C. R. Brewin (2003).[54]*

In some cases, recovered memories have been authenticated by external sources whereas in other cases, there is no proof regarding the veracity of the alleged sexual contact.[45,46] Although there is little rigorous research on this question, it has been suggested that most "recovered" memories have been triggered spontaneously by later life events that resembled the initial trauma and not by participation in psychotherapy.[49,55,56]

Some patients who claim to have regained traumatic memories of this nature have confronted their parents whom they have come to regard as perpetrators of childhood sexual trauma, sometimes taking these parents to court for alleged abuses. Sometimes the accused parents vehemently deny that such events ever occurred and maintain that such "recovered traumatic memories" are really emblematic of a "false memory syndrome" manufactured in the course of therapy.[49,53]

Researchers generally agree that:[49–60]

- ► Memory, especially childhood memory, is fallible but not necessarily incorrect.
- ► Documented traumatic events are sometimes forgotten.
- ► There is adequate proof of a few cases in which forgotten traumatic memories were later "recovered," but it is not known whether this is an extremely rare or frequent event.

Clinicians need to familiarize themselves with the complexity, fallibility, and reconstructive nature of human memory.[49]

Though this issue remains controversial, there is general agreement that clinicians should emphasize to patients the fallibility of memory and avoid aggressive techniques to "retrieve" inaccessible memories. They should also desist from suggesting that a patient's current symptoms are an indication of a previous traumatic experience for which no recollection exists.[49]

What Are the Major Personal Issues for Clinicians Treating Those with PTSD?

Clinicians treating individuals with PTSD must deal with how the patient's reports of human suffering impact the clinician personally. Specific issues to note include:

► Therapeutic neutrality vs. advocacy
► *Secondary traumatization*
► *Countertransference*
► Clinician self-care

Therapeutic Neutrality vs. Advocacy

Trauma work challenges the traditional psychotherapeutic principle of clinician *neutrality* because so many people seeking help have suffered from abusive violence, state-sponsored terrorism, or other man-made catastrophes. It is only natural that clinicians' feelings about such injustices are mobilized and channeled into advocacy activities to prevent such human suffering in the future. However, advocacy can undermine therapy.[61] For example, the clinician should never assume the role of rescuer for a specific patient. When a clinician intervenes directly to confront a problem that the patient seems unable to address, it implies that the patient cannot cope with problems without assistance. The more the clinician's words and deeds suggest that the patient is helpless, the more disempowered the patient becomes. Such clinician behavior perpetuates patient beliefs about being personally incompetent and that the world is overwhelming.

In contrast, clinicians can and should act as advocates for patients in obtaining services requiring a professional referral. Such advocacy might include dealing with local, state, or federal agencies to gain access to community support or victim assistance programs. Military mental health professionals, especially during war, face a uniquely complicated challenge with regard to their stance toward their patients. Although their major objective is to diagnose and treat servicemen and servicewomen as do their civilian counterparts, their primary client objective is to maintain the fighting force at optimal strength. As a result, civilian priorities to safeguard privacy and confidentiality are sometimes trumped by the necessity of informing Military Command about unfitness for duty of a patient who does not want such information divulged. In other words, military mental health professionals are constantly challenged by the necessity of achieving a proper balance between patient privacy and Military Command's need to know about the functional capacity of the troops.

secondary traumatization—feelings, personal distress, and symptoms sometimes evoked in people who live with an individual with PTSD

countertransference—the clinician's personal psychological reaction to something the patient said or did

neutrality—a therapeutic stance in which clinicians reveal as little of themselves as possible so that thoughts, memories, and feelings generated during therapy come from the patient's intrapsychic processes rather than from an interpersonal relationship between patient and clinician

Vicarious Traumatization

Vicarious traumatization can cause severe personal distress among clinicians and can impair their professional judgment and performance so that their therapeutic efforts become unhelpful or even detrimental to their patients.[62,63]

Working with patients who have suffered trauma is difficult. Patients' powerful stories often generate intense emotions within clinicians who may despair because they are powerless to protect patients (especially children) or feel guilty that they were not personally exposed to such horrors.

Vicarious traumatization can produce a number of inappropriate behaviors that compromise therapy or may even disturb the clinician on a personal level, such as engaging in ill-advised rescue attempts or becoming personally involved in the patient's daily life.[60]

Clinicians may become so overwhelmed by the traumatic experiences reported by their patients that they have intrusive recollections and nightmares about such material, which in turn activate avoidant/numbing behavior, guilt, feelings of powerlessness, rescue fantasies, doubting, denial, intellectualization, constricted affect, dissociation, minimization, or avoidance of traumatic material. This process has been called "vicarious traumatization" or "compassion fatigue."[62,63]

Countertransference

A variety of credible resources address countertransference in the context of PTSD.[61,64,65]

Since more than half of all American men and women will be exposed to at least one traumatic event during their lives, it is likely that many mental health professionals will also have been traumatized—among whom, some undoubtedly will have developed PTSD.[1]

Countertransference, a psychoanalytic term, refers to personal memories and feelings elicited from the clinician by the patient in the course of therapy. Whereas secondary traumatization refers to a psychological response that might occur among clinicians who have never experienced trauma, countertransference applies to situations in which patient recollections trigger intrusive recollections in the clinicians, themselves, of personal traumatic or other significant experiences. Countertransference can significantly interfere with therapy if the elicited feelings are either unrecognized or unresolved.

Countertransference most likely occurs when the similarities between patient and clinician experiences are sufficient to trigger the clinician's intrusive recollections, avoidant/numbing, or hyperarousal symptoms as well as other intrapsychic and interpersonal issues.

An important variation on this theme is the countertransference that occurs when clinicians themselves are attempting to cope with the same catastrophic stresses as their patients. For example, clinicians working in a war zone or natural disaster area are also personally affected by the catastrophic stresses for which their patients seek treatment. Under such circumstances, it is suggested that clinicians seek support, supervision, and possibly treatment for their own posttraumatic distress if they expect to be able to help others.

Clinician Self-Care

Whether due to *vicarious traumatization* or countertransference, disturbing feelings and thoughts can impair both the personal mental health and the professional performance of clinicians treating individuals with PTSD. Clinicians may find themselves trapped in a vicious cycle in which the more symptomatic, maladaptive, and ineffective they become, the more they minimize this state of affairs and plunge themselves into their work. Unfortunately, under such circumstances clinicians most desperately need (but frequently fail or refuse to seek) the supervision or assistance of their colleagues.

Recognizing these occupational hazards or personal difficulties is only the first step. Clinicians must make a conscious, sustained, and systematic effort to prevent or remedy vicarious traumatization or countertransference. This can be accomplished through professional and personal self-care activities, such as:[66,67]

- ▶ Having regular supervision
- ▶ Developing a supportive environment at work
- ▶ Placing limits on one's caseload—especially with respect to the number of trauma cases
- ▶ Maintaining boundaries between personal and professional activities
- ▶ Prioritizing personal, marital, and family commitments in relation to professional commitments
- ▶ Engaging in regular exercise, hobbies, friendships, emotional enrichment, artistic endeavors, and spiritual pursuits

vicarious traumatization— feelings, personal distress, and symptoms that are sometimes evoked in clinicians working with PTSD patients

Key Concepts for Chapter 3

1. It is important for clinicians to take a careful history to determine what causes a patient to seek help for chronic PTSD symptoms at a particular time. The timing usually relates to some abrupt change in the patient's life that has disrupted his or her ability to cope with both the symptoms and daily demands.

2. Clinicians may need to address psychiatric emergencies, substance abuse, or a marital/familial/ workplace crisis prior to initiating treatment for PTSD.

3. Determining the best treatment approach for a patient with PTSD involves consideration of combined treatments, comorbidity, cross-cultural differences in how symptoms are expressed and dealt with, controversial recovered memories, and the patient's emotional safety, as well as whether a longer, more comprehensive treatment plan should be considered for those who might have "complex PTSD."

4. Trauma-focused therapy explores the memories of the trauma in depth to facilitate healing and uses techniques that range from cognitive behavioral to psychodynamic approaches.

5. Supportive therapy focuses on building coping skills and solving problems to enhance functioning and regain a sense of control over one's life.

6. Although untested, simultaneously treating comorbid alcohol and substance abuse/dependence with PTSD appears to be preferable as each disorder exacerbates the other.

7. Patient reports of human suffering and catastrophe can impact clinicians in ways that compromise their therapeutic neutrality, cause them to suffer guilt and feelings of powerlessness that can lead to inappropriate behaviors, or invoke personally painful memories or unresolved feelings (countertransference).

8. Clinicians should attend to their own professional and personal care by creating a supportive work environment with regular supervision, establishing personal boundaries, and limiting their caseload to maintain a healthy personal/professional balance.

Chapter 4
Psychological Treatments for PTSD

This chapter answers the following questions:

▶ **What Specific Psychosocial Treatments Are Available for Adults with PTSD?**— This section reviews the treatment approach and effectiveness of psychoeducation, individual psychotherapy, and group therapy for adult patients with PTSD.

▶ **What Psychosocial Treatments Are Available for Children and Adolescents with PTSD?**—This section covers the treatment approaches used specifically for children and adolescents with PTSD.

What Specific Psychosocial Treatments Are Available for Adults with PTSD?

THERE are many psychosocial treatments for PTSD, all of which share the general stages and focus of treatment issues discussed in Chapter 3. Treatments generally fall into three categories:

1. **Psychoeducation**—Designed to help patients understand the nature of PTSD and its impact on their lives

2. **Individual Psychotherapy**—Geared to treat specific symptoms of PTSD through, typically, one of three approaches: cognitive behavioral therapy CBT), eye movement desensitization reprocessing (EMDR), or psychodynamic psychotherapy (see pages 43–54)

3. **Group Therapy**— Structured to treat PTSD in a group setting that promotes a connection among members through shared experiences, which can foster adaptive coping strategies, reduce symptoms, and/or help patients derive meaning from the traumatic experience (see pages 54–58)

In this chapter, efficacy research results are covered immediately following the discussion of the approach for each individual therapy. General efficacy information appears with the general overview of each category of treatment.

Psychoeducation

It is relatively easy to move from a comprehensive diagnostic assessment (see Chapter 2) into a psychoeducational phase of treatment by showing patients how their various reexperiencing, avoidance/numbing, and arousal symptoms fit into a coherent syndrome. Patients need to understand that they are not losing their minds (as many of them genuinely fear to be the case); that their constellation of symptoms has a specific name; that many other people have suffered in a similar way after exposure to

Psychoeducation is generally not considered an effective treatment for PTSD (or ASD) on its own.

catastrophic stress; and, most importantly, that there are effective treatments for PTSD.

There have been few rigorous clinical trials testing the efficacy of psychoeducation as a stand-alone PTSD treatment. Two of the best were done with U.K. Royal Navy personnel and Turkish survivors of the Marmara earthquake. In the first (which did not assess PTSD outcomes, per se), a trauma risk management program significantly improved attitudes about stress and help-seeking behavior among British sailors.[68] In the second, earthquake survivors randomized to a combined treatment with both psychoeducation and medication showed significantly greater reduction in PTSD symptoms than those who received either psychoeducation or medication alone[69]. Two other randomized trials showed that self-help information, provided to acutely stressed patients seeking emergency room treatment shortly after an accident, failed to prevent the later development of PTSD.[70,71]

Despite the paucity of solid research in this area, there is a strong consensus among clinicians that it is a very important component of any therapeutic approach. In fact, most cognitive-behavioral treatments have a specific psychoeducational component during early treatment sessions.

Psychoeducation may also be especially useful as a societal and community intervention utilizing the mass media to promote resilience and ameliorate distress for the population at large following terrorism or mass casualties (see Chapter 6).[13]

Psychoeducation to Initiate Therapeutic Activity

The benefits of psychoeducational intervention appear to make it a very important and productive component of any treatment approach.

> *Accurate information helps patients recognize that they are not losing their minds; that there is no stigma attached to this kind of all-too-human response to an overwhelming experience; and that they do not have to be ashamed of having PTSD symptoms.*

- ► Achieve Normalization—Just telling people that the nature of their posttraumatic emotional disturbance is no different from the experience of millions of men, women, and children exposed to similar stresses engenders a profound sense of relief in most people.

- ► Remove Self-Blame and Self-Doubt—Telling patients that PTSD is fundamentally about being in the wrong place at the wrong time, and being overwhelmed by a stressor with which no one could have been expected to cope, is a powerful message that most patients can hear readily. It is an important message that helps remove self-blame and self-doubt, because most humans do not face these overwhelming events as they would have wished, despite tales of heroes and heroines glorified throughout history.

▶ Correct Misunderstandings—Another important benefit of psychoeducation is that the PTSD model helps people understand disturbing behavior that they may have interpreted erroneously. For example, a wife married to a serviceman who was recently deployed to a war zone, who blames herself for the sexual and emotional withdrawal of her recently returned spouse, will learn that this is not a personal rejection but rather the expression of her husband's PTSD avoidance/numbing symptoms due to war-zone trauma. Reframing the problem in this way can focus treatment on the root of the problem and often save a marriage before things deteriorate beyond repair.

▶ Enhance Clinician Credibility—The final advantage of psychoeducation is that it quickly lets patients know that the clinician understands their problem at its most fundamental level. It is a rapid and effective communication that the clinician deserves trust and is qualified to treat them, helping them make sense of their disturbing and disruptive symptoms.

Community Psychoeducation: Three Examples

After the Loma Prieta earthquake in California in 1989, local mental health centers immediately distributed age-appropriate pamphlets and coloring books in English and Spanish to help residents understand normal post-disaster symptoms and when to ask for help.

After the 9/11 World Trade Center attacks, New York's Project Liberty utilized 30-second TV commercials, radio announcements, printed brochures, a cost-free "800" crisis line, and a Web site (see Chapter 6 for more information on Project Liberty).

Currently, the U.S. Army routinely provides BATTLEMIND training, which is a psychoeducational intervention provided to service members at the time they return home from the war zone. The basic premise is that the military mindset that enabled them to function effectively in the war zones of Iraq and Afghanistan is maladaptive at home and needs to be recalibrated. Potential problem areas such as inappropriate aggression, emotional detachment, hypervigilance, and aggressive driving are each targeted in one of the BATTLEMIND modules. Initial evaluations suggest that this approach has made a significant difference for returning army personnel who have received it.[72]

Psychoeducation Through Peer Counseling

One type of psychoeducation, peer counseling, is a powerful group process for PTSD sufferers similar to Alcoholics Anonymous. Peer counseling provides a context of peer support within which participants can take control of their lives by seeking more effective ways to cope with their PTSD symptoms.

Another benefit of peer counseling is that there is no authority figure such as a doctoral-level clinician. Instead, everyone is an equal authority based on his or her own personal experience. Participants are simultaneously patients and therapists, able to give and receive assistance to one another through honest disclosure and genuine response in the context of absolute trust and confidentiality.

Rape crisis centers and battered women's shelters use peer counseling. Counselors who have survived their own sexual trauma and/or domestic violence have subsequently found meaning in their suffering and have transformed their personal suffering into knowledge that they use to help others cope with similar experiences. It is reaffirming to know that others have been able to pick up the pieces of their shattered lives and move on to a future that is gratifying and productive.

A recent addition to peer counseling approaches in the United States has been a Vet-to-Vet program for returnees from Iraq and Afghanistan. Veterans who are experiencing postdeployment problems at home, in the workplace, or in the community may seek support from other veterans who have faced the same challenges. The advantages of this approach are that the peer counselor has experiential authenticity, having been deployed in the past. The help-seeking veteran does not have to overcome the stigma of requesting formal mental health treatment, and all interactions are strictly confidential. Although this program has been extremely useful, it is limited in what it can realistically accomplish. The challenge of peer counseling is to convince veterans with clinically significant problems to seek formal treatment from mental health professionals, when it is indicated.

Since peer counseling is a consumer-driven approach that excludes professional clinicians, it does not lend itself to scientific research protocols in which some patients receive active treatment while others do not. It is clear that people who continue to participate in peer counseling do so because they find the format and support beneficial.

From the Patient's Perspective

Had my fifth session of exposure treatment today. It's hard to admit how scared I was at first. After all, Dr. Owen wanted me to imagine I was back in the car and to go through the whole accident detail by detail. I was terrified and sure that I'd fall apart. But she was patient. Didn't rush me. And backed off when I started to lose it. Before I knew it, I could really let myself begin to remember what happened. And the more I did it, the easier it got, and the less upset I became.

I'm not there yet. It's still very painful to keep bringing back all that stuff about the accident. But I am getting stronger, and I have another five sessions to go.

Individual Psychotherapies

Clinicians primarily use three different types of individual psychotherapy to treat PTSD:

1. Cognitive Behavioral Therapy (CBT)—Based on principles of learning theory and cognitive psychology. A number of different CBT approaches will be described. The two most powerful CBT treatments are Prolonged Exposure (PE) and Cognitive Processing Therapy (CPT).

2. Eye Movement Desensitization and Reprocessing (EMDR)—Based on the theory that rapid eye movements reprogram the brain's processing of traumatic memories.

3. Psychodynamic Psychotherapy Based on the theory that symptoms of PTSD result from repressed memories of the traumatic event and that the patient's insight into those memories and their impact on symptoms will help restore psychological balance.

Cognitive-Behavioral Therapy (CBT)

Given the fact that PTSD develops when exposure to an overwhelming stimulus (the criterion A_1 event) elicits a profound emotional reaction (the criterion A_2 response), it is understandable why learning and conditioning models have provided such a powerful conceptual approach to PTSD. The sudden, intense anxiety experienced by Mary T. in response to the sight or sound of a large tractor-trailer truck is an excellent example of fear conditioning. Here, the traumatic stimulus (the truck) automatically evokes the posttraumatic emotional response (fear, helplessness, and horror). The intensity of this emotional reaction provokes avoidant behaviors that will reduce the emotional impact of such a stimulus. Successful reduction of intrusion and hyperarousal symptoms by such avoidance increases the likelihood that avoidant behaviors will be repeated in the future because they provide short-term relief.

There are more published well-controlled studies on CBT (especially PE and CPT) than on any other PTSD treatment.[73] Furthermore, the magnitude of treatment effects appears greater with CBT than with any other therapeutic approach. As a result, all clinical practice guidelines for PTSD have endorsed CBT as the most effective treatment. These various practice guidelines have been developed by the American Psychiatric Association (APA), the American Academy of Child and Adolescent Psychiatry (AACAP), the International Society for Traumatic Stress Studies (ISTSS), the British National Institute for Clinical Excellence (NICE), the Australian National Health Medical Research Council (NHMRC), and the American government's joint guidelines from the Departments of Veterans Affairs and Defense (VA/DoD).[33–38]

From a cognitive psychological perspective, trauma exposure is thought to evoke erroneous automatic thoughts about the environment (as dangerous and threatening) and about oneself (as helpless and incompetent). CBT directly confronts such PTSD-related distortions in thinking.

Various CBT approaches seek to attack these conditioned responses and automatic thoughts with different techniques. The ultimate goal is to normalize the abnormal feelings, thoughts, and behaviors exhibited by individuals with PTSD. CBT has proven to be the best treatment for PTSD in the current published literature; CBT techniques are sometimes used in combination with one another. Figure 4.1, on page 45, provides an at-a-glance introduction to CBT techniques.

Prolonged Exposure (PE) Therapy

Clinicians ask patients receiving *imaginal exposure* to narrate the traumatic event. If numerous traumatic episodes exist (as with survivors of recurrent child abuse, domestic violence, war trauma, or torture), the clinician asks patients to construct narratives about the worst events they clearly remember. The clinician prompts patients to close their eyes and visualize (imagine) what happened while repeating the narrative several times during a single session. Initially, patients experience great anxiety as they begin to imagine themselves back in the traumatic situation. They are asked to rate their level of subjective distress

---

In general, cognitive-behavioral therapy is the most proven treatment for PTSD to date, although differences exist among various CBT approaches (as shown here). CBT treatments involve carefully scripted treatment manuals and usually require nine to 16 sessions. See individual approaches for specific efficacy studies to date.[74]

imaginal exposure—
systematically assisting trauma survivors to confront distressing trauma memories though the use of mental imagery

Figure 4.1 Cognitive Behavioral Techniques Used in PTSD Treatment[64–66]

CBT Technique	Treatment Focus
Prolonged Exposure (PE) Therapy	Disconnecting the overwhelming sense of fear from trauma memories; extinguishing PTSD fear conditioning
Cognitive Therapy	Reframing thoughts and beliefs generated from the traumatic event, which impede current coping skills
Cognitive Processing Therapy (CPT)	Addressing both the erroneous cognitions and emotional responses resulting from trauma exposure
Stress Inoculation Training (SIT)	Anxiety management to increase coping skills for current situations
Internet-Based Therapies	Exposure and cognitive restructuring through a protocol-driven CBT treatment accessed via the Internet
Imagery Rehearsal Therapy	Changing disturbing traumatic nightmares by rehearsing a "new dream"
Biofeedback and Relaxation Training	Anxiety management to help patients master overwhelming anxiety feelings and physiological reactions elicited by a trauma reminder
Dialectical Behavior Therapy (DBT)	Treating borderline personality disorder, a syndrome often associated with PTSD and complex PTSD

every 10 minutes on a 10–100 *Subjective Units of Distress Scale* (SUDS), where 10 is no distress and 100 is the most fear/helplessness/horror they have ever experienced. Distress levels are usually in the 70–90 range during initial imaginal exposure sessions. However, through repeated exposure to the traumatic memory, patients experience a progressive reduction in distress levels so that they may fall to the 10–20 range by the end of a single session and remain at negligible levels by the end of an 8- to 10-session exposure therapy treatment. Following successful exposure treatment, patients can confront traumatic memories without having the recollections trigger intrusive and/or hyperarousal PTSD symptoms.

When ready, patients are encouraged, as part of a homework assignment, to confront situations associated with their traumatic experiences in the context of *in-vivo exposure*.[30,73–77]

The mechanism of action of PE is thought to be through extinction of negative emotions (fear, anxiety, sadness, guilt) associated with traumatic reminders. The protocol, by which patients are repeatedly exposed to their own individualized trauma stimuli until their SUDS levels have been persistently reduced, is directly comparable to psychological laboratory extinction paradigms following fear conditioning. As a result, it is possible to carry out laboratory research that has direct relevance to PE. For example, animal research with D-cycloserine (see below) raised the possibility that such an approach might have clinical benefit.[40]

Subjective Units of Distress Scale—a scale ranging from 10 to 100 with 10 being the least anxiety provoking and 100 being the most anxiety provoking; the SUDS scoring system allows the patient to express exactly how upsetting or distressing certain stimuli are in comparison to other anxiety experiences

in-vivo exposure—patients practice techniques learned in therapy in the environment that represents their most-feared situation

PE may not be for everyone; some patients are either not ready or not willing to confront traumatic reminders and the intense anxiety provoked by this technique.

An important variant of PE is Virtual Reality (VR) exposure therapy, which uses a computer-generated visual, auditory, and kinesthetic model of the patient's own traumatic experience during the therapy session. There is a popular misconception that VR is a unique treatment unto itself. Actually, VR is nothing more than PE treatment provided with the aid of a multimedia delivery system. A VR approach for American veterans of the war in Iraq, called "Virtual Iraq," exposes patients to desert scenarios in which (for example) the detonation of improvised explosive devices (IEDs) is displayed. Virtual Iraq has been used effectively with military personnel and veterans alike.[78] At this time it is not known how VR compares with conventional PE. What is known is that both treatments are extremely effective.

A very exciting recent development has been combining PE with the medication D-cycloserine (DCS). As discussed in Chapter 5, there is evidence that patients receiving PE plus DCS improve more quickly than those receiving PE alone.

Efficacy—PE has consistently proven superior to supportive counseling or untreated patients monitored while on a "waiting list" for therapy. It is equal in efficacy to other forms of CBT treatment; results have shown 60 to 70 percent improvement in all three PTSD symptom clusters, with improvements generally maintained 6 and 12 months later. In one important study, improvement from PE was sustained for five years.[73,77–81]

Cognitive Therapy

Cognitive therapy addresses thoughts and beliefs generated by the traumatic event rather than conditioned emotional responses addressed by exposure therapy.[73,76–79,82,83] This approach focuses on how individuals with PTSD have interpreted the traumatic event with respect to their appraisals about the world and themselves. For example, those who have been overwhelmed by a catastrophic stressor typically perceive the world as dangerous and themselves as incompetent. As a result, PTSD patients see themselves as perennial victims powerless to cope with life and take charge of their personal destiny. Such a belief system then becomes a hard-wired, self-fulfilling prophecy.

PE, with or without cognitive therapy, has been tested with survivors of a great variety of traumatic events, including sexual assault, war-zone exposure, or childhood sexual abuse.

Clinicians often combine cognitive therapy with exposure therapy to work on both conditioned emotional responses and automatic dysfunctional thoughts. One somewhat different approach for combining cognitive and exposure therapy is cognitive processing therapy (CPT).

> **Case Study Notes**
>
> Mary T.'s persistent inability to overcome her PTSD symptoms and resume her life as before has destroyed her confidence in herself. She has come to think of herself as a failure, someone unable to cope with even minor stressors. Because of this pervasive sense of personal inadequacy, she is easily overwhelmed and unable to perform routine tasks. It is a vicious circle since the more she fails to perform, the more she feels inadequate, and the more she finds the world overwhelming.

In cognitive therapy, the first step is to identify dysfunctional automatic thoughts (such as Mary's thoughts about herself) and to understand that, although originally developed from the trauma, these thoughts currently hinder adaptive functioning. Second, the therapy focuses on challenging and disputing these beliefs by examining evidence for or against them. Third, treatment focuses on correcting such erroneous thoughts with more accurate information or replacing automatic, dysfunctional thoughts with more realistic, evidence-based, and adaptive beliefs. Successful cognitive therapy creates an accurate appraisal of:

▶ Situations perceived as either safe or dangerous rather than automatically perceiving all external events as dangerous

> **Case Study Notes**
>
> Mary needs to learn that there is nothing inherently dangerous about trucks or about driving a car. She needs to separate the specific tragic circumstances of her personal trauma from the trauma-related generalizations that currently make her afraid to travel on the highway.

▶ One's own strengths and weaknesses in different situations rather than an automatic belief that one is personally incompetent and unable to cope with life's challenges

> **Case Study Notes**
>
> Mary needs to understand that what happened during the accident was not due to a failure on her part and to learn that her current immobility is due to PTSD and not due to her own personal inadequacies.

Efficacy—Several studies comparing cognitive therapy with PE (alone and in combination) found equal effectiveness, producing 60 to 70 percent improvement in PTSD symptoms. Additionally, these individual or combined approaches outperformed relaxation therapy.[73,77,79,84,85]

Cognitive Processing Therapy (CPT)

CPT also uses written narratives to address both the emotional and cognitive consequences of trauma exposure so that patients can access and process the natural emotions that have been distorted and obscured by their personal interpretations of the traumatic event.[73,86,87]

According to CPT theory, negative belief systems that a person generates following a trauma (e.g., "I am powerless," "I am inadequate," "The world is a dangerous place") make it impossible to process normal emotional reactions to the catastrophic event (e.g., sadness and fear). This happens because the trauma survivor is preoccupied with inappropriate and intolerable emotions (e.g., guilt and shame) evolving from erroneous beliefs and interpretations about the traumatic experience. By confronting distorted traumatic memories, patients challenge/modify these erroneous beliefs, thereby dissipating inappropriate emotions.

CPT has both cognitive and exposure components. The exposure component differs from exposure therapy because the narratives are written by patients rather than elicited orally by the clinician. The written format gives the CPT patient more control over the pace and intensity of disclosure than is the case in exposure treatment. Recent dismantling studies have attempted to evaluate the relative contribution of the cognitive versus exposure component to CPT. In one study, CPT that included only the cognitive component was found to be just as effective as CPT that included both cognitive and exposure components.

Case Study Notes

Mary T.'s inappropriate feelings of guilt about the accident and shame about her current feelings of inadequacy have dominated her feelings about the traumatic event. They have prevented her from normal grieving about the loss of her husband, her marriage, her future, and the person she was before the accident. Psychological recovery depends upon moving beyond trauma-engendered cognitive distortions and inappropriate emotions so that she can freely process normal emotions (e.g., sadness and fear) that have been inaccessible up to this point.

Efficacy—In studies conducted with patients having rape-related PTSD, CPT performed as well as PE initially and 6 and 12 months after. All patients had significant reduction in all three PTSD symptom clusters, and none continued to meet PTSD diagnostic criteria at the six-month follow-up. A recent, very large study comparing both approaches demonstrated equal effectiveness. Furthermore, remission of PTSD following either PE or CPT persisted for five years [73,80,86]

Stress Inoculation Training (SIT)

Originally adapted for treating rape victims, SIT provides PTSD patients with a repertoire of tools and skills they can utilize to control anxiety elicited either by trauma-related stimuli or during threatening situations.[88,89] It combines a variety of anxiety management techniques including education, muscle relaxation training, and biofeedback (breathing) retraining (see page 50). In addition, SIT utilizes the following:[73]

> *SIT aims to reduce avoidance behavior through anxiety reduction and to foster a sense of personal competence.*

▶ Social skills training—Clinicians help patients increase specific interpersonal skills necessary for positive relationships. This includes assertiveness training.

▶ Role-playing—Clinicians and patients practice responses to specific situations.

▶ Distraction techniques (e.g., thought stopping)— Clinicians teach patients to yell "stop" to themselves each time certain thoughts start.

▶ Positive thinking and self-talk—Clinicians teach patients how to replace negative with positive thoughts, especially when confronting stressful situations.

Efficacy—Four studies on women with rape-related PTSD or male or female motor vehicle accident survivors tested SIT alone or in combination with PE. In all cases, results from SIT were equal to those from PE, producing a 60 to 70 percent reduction in PTSD symptom severity. Three-month follow-up assessments showed substantial improvement in one study and improvement slightly better with PE than SIT in another study. More recently, SIT has been incorporated in an Internet-based CBT protocol (see below) for U.S. military personnel (e.g., DE-STRESS), which has proven effective.[81,86,90,91]

> *Given the avoidance behavior that characterizes PTSD, growing Internet access worldwide, and the shortage of skilled CBT clinicians, Internet approaches have much to recommend them for addressing the spectrum of posttraumatic distress, from acute stress reactions to PTSD*

Internet Approaches

Internet approaches modify standard CBT components (especially CPT psychoeducation, exposure, and cognitive therapies as well as SIT anxiety management). One was originally tested in the Netherlands and named Interapy. It involves 10 sessions (twice a week for five weeks). Patients submit essays (approximately 450 words) to a Web site and receive clinician feedback. Major components are exposure, "self confrontation," and cognitive reappraisal, much along the lines of CPT. Since that time there have been other successful trials of Web-based CBT treatments with American civilian and military personnel. An advantage of Internet treatment, especially for military personnel worried about confidentiality and the stigma of seeking treatment in a mental health clinic, is that it ensures privacy.

Efficacy—There have been two controlled trials of Interapy, one with students and one with 184 Dutch participants, who reported mild to severe posttraumatic symptoms. Neither study included formal PTSD diagnostic assessment; however, researchers observed a 50 percent or greater improvement in PTSD, depression, and other symptoms.[92,93] Two additional trials have been reported with American civilians and servicemembers. Although promising, they were less successful than the Dutch trials.[94,95] More research is needed for this exciting treatment option.

Imagery Rehearsal Therapy (IRT)

IRT was developed to decrease the traumatic nightmares central to PTSD, reduce insomnia, and decrease PTSD symptom severity. IRT treatment consists of three weekly sessions in which patients learn cognitive-behavioral techniques for replacing unpleasant images with pleasant ones. It is often delivered in a group format. The specific components of IRT are (a) psychoeducation about nightmares and PTSD; (b) anxiety management skills; (c) cognitive restructuring; (d) sleep hygiene; and (e) focused use of pleasant imagery to replace negative imagery in recurrent traumatic nightmares. Patients focus on a single intolerable nightmare and are instructed to "change the nightmare" in any way they wish. Then they rehearse this new dream five to 20 minutes every day.

Efficacy—Four randomized IRT trials with crime victims, sexually abused adolescent girls and women, and Vietnam veterans have reported 50 to 60 percent reduction in nightmare frequency and overall PTSD symptom severity.[96-98] Further testing is needed, but IRT appears to be a promising, unique approach for PTSD patients experiencing nightmares.

Biofeedback and Relaxation Training

Biofeedback is a process to reduce tension and anxiety in which the patient is given information about her or his own physiological processes. For example, the patient is given continuous feedback about heart rate or muscle tension and learns to consciously control these processes. Success is demonstrated by reductions in heart rate, muscle tension, or other physiological processes. Relaxation training is a treatment in which patients learn to relax their musculature through breathing and meditation-like tensing and untensing exercises, often assisted by audiotapes. Learning to induce muscle relaxation at will is used as a technique to control anxiety, when it occurs.

Efficacy—Biofeedback and relaxation training are ineffective stand-alone treatments, but they are usually included with other anxiety management techniques in CBT approaches, such as stress inoculation training (SIT) (reviewed on page 49).[73]

Dialectical Behavior Therapy (DBT)[29,44]

DBT is a comprehensive CBT approach designed specifically for patients with *borderline personality disorder*, emotion dysregulation, self-destructive and suicidal behavior, impulsive behavior, substance abuse, and for other difficult-to-treat patients too unstable to adhere to other treatments. Since DBT candidates often have significant trauma histories and often meet diagnostic criteria for PTSD or complex PTSD, this option may be appropriate for the initial stabilization (e.g., establishing trust and safety) phase of PTSD treatment.

DBT patients acquire skills to reduce chronic impulsive behavior marked by chaotic life problems, suicidal behavior, emotional liability, substance abuse, binge eating, and frequent hospitalizations. DBT is characterized by a balanced and flexible approach to therapy based on a strong patient-clinician relationship through which problem behaviors are explicitly addressed.

Efficacy—There have been no clinical trials of DBT for PTSD. Advocates of DBT for complicated PTSD patients argue that these individuals are too impulsive and disorganized to comply with a standard CBT protocol until they have been clinically stabilized through DBT. A number of reports describe moderate improvement for such complex patients receiving DBT with respect to suicidal, self-mutilating, impulsive, self-damaging, and binge-eating behaviors.[29,44,100,101]

Eye Movement Desensitization and Reprocessing (EMDR)

EMDR is an effective treatment for PTSD. Based on positive data from clinical trials, EMDR is ranked as a first-line treatment in most clinical practice guidelines.[102] Proponents of the treatment believe that *saccadic eye movements* (or some other repetitive motor activity) reprogram brain function so that the emotional impact of a trauma can be finally and completely resolved.[103,104] When conducting EMDR, the clinician instructs the patient to imagine a painful, traumatic memory and an associated negative cognition (e.g., guilt, shame). Then the patient is asked to articulate an incompatible positive cognition (e.g., personal worth, self-efficacy, trustworthiness). The clinician has the patient contemplate the traumatic memory while visually focusing on the rapid movement of the clinician's fingers. After

borderline personality disorder—a personality disorder characterized by extreme instabilities fluctuating between normal functioning and psychic disability

See page 41 for more information on establishing trust and safety.

For a specific model for integrating DBT with prolonged exposure for PTSD, see C. B. Becker and C. Zayfert.[99]

saccadic eye movements—rapid intermittent eye movement, such as that which occurs when the eyes fix on one point after another in the visual field

each set of 10–12 eye movements, the clinician asks the patient to rate the strength of both the distressing memory and his or her belief in the positive cognition.

Despite the name of this therapy, research evidence suggests that eye movements do not appear necessary for EMDR to work.[102,105] In published studies comparing conventional EMDR to EMDR minus eye movements, patients who received EMDR minus eye movements did just as well as those who received conventional EMDR. Therefore, it is difficult to substantiate that eye movements form the crucial ingredient in EMDR and even more difficult to defend the hypothesis that EMDR reprograms the brain's processing of traumatic memories.

Frankly, it is less important how EMDR works than the fact that it does work very effectively. Since eye movements don't seem to be the key therapeutic ingredient, more research is needed to understand the actual mechanism of action. Some theorists believe that EMDR is actually a unique variant of exposure therapy, with a novel protocol for exposing patients to their own traumatic material. It may also be especially useful for individuals who cannot bring themselves to talk about their traumatic experiences, as in PE or CPT, but who can permit themselves to think about the traumatic event in the safety of a therapist's office. In practice, EMDR does have some unique components that may account for its appeal among clinicians as well as its therapeutic efficacy. Most notable is the practice of having patients select the traumatic material, which they process in their own ways and at their own paces—in contrast to other approaches.[106]

Efficacy—EMDR appears to be more effective than no treatment among patients assigned to a wait list. It is also superior to psychodynamic, relaxation, or supportive therapies.

Several studies have shown that, in comparison with wait-list patients (who show little improvement), approximately two-thirds of those receiving EMDR no longer met PTSD diagnostic criteria.[102,107,108,111,112]

Published results indicate that following treatment, 50 to 77 percent of those receiving EMDR no longer met criteria for the PTSD diagnosis, in comparison to 20 to 50 percent of patients receiving supportive therapy, relaxation therapy or treatment-as-usual.[106–110]

EMDR proponents argue that their treatment is not only as effective as CBT, but that it is shorter and better tolerated by patients.

Results are mixed regarding the relative efficacy of EMDR and CBT. Four studies specifically comparing EMDR with exposure therapy generally found the two therapies equally effective. EMDR proponents assert that EMDR is more efficient because fewer trials are needed, while PE proponents argue that PE produces better and longer-lasting outcomes.[102,111–115] Four meta-analyses have also concluded that both treatments are equally effective.[116–119]

Psychodynamic Psychotherapy

For more than 100 years, clinicians have used psychodynamic psychotherapy to treat posttraumatic disorders. Psychodynamic theory focuses on *psychic balance*, which sometimes requires the patient to force intolerable thoughts and feelings out of conscious awareness through the process called *repression*. However, these now-unconscious traumatic memories are still powerful enough to become expressed as symptoms, such as PTSD's intrusion, avoidant/numbing, and hyperarousal symptoms.[120]

Psychodynamic treatment seeks to understand the context of the traumatic memories and the defensive processes through which the unconscious transforms repressed memories into the maladaptive symptoms that initially drive treatment. According to psychoanalytic theory, simply focusing on symptom reduction can achieve little as long as repressed memories remain.[120]

A new, healthier balance must be achieved by confronting unconscious processes that have repressed the memories and produced maladaptive compromises (e.g., symptoms). As these feelings, behaviors, and memories are explored, patients gain insight or understanding of how their repressed memories (along with associated thoughts and feelings) have been transformed into their current symptoms. This awareness ideally enables patients to exercise more control over the repression defense and thereby achieve symptom reduction.

Psychodynamic treatments vary from 10–20 sessions to open-ended treatment lasting many years. Longer psychodynamic treatments seek to create a fundamental change in psychic balance, while briefer forms (12–15 sessions) seek to foster improved self-understanding and ego-strength.

Brief Psychodynamic Psychotherapy (BPP)

This type of therapy, conducted within 12–15 sessions, focuses on the traumatic event itself. Through the retelling of the trauma story to a calm, empathetic, compassionate, and nonjudgmental clinician, the patient achieves a greater sense of *self-cohesion*, develops more adaptive defenses and coping strategies, and successfully modulates the intense emotions that emerge during therapy.[124] While working through the traumatic memories, the clinician also addresses the linkage between posttraumatic distress and current life stress. Patients learn to identify current life situations and environmental triggers that set off traumatic memories and exacerbate PTSD symptoms.

Efficacy—Because psychodynamic treatment focuses primarily on psychic processes rather than psychiatric symptoms, there

psychic balance—a dynamic equilibrium state between those thoughts, feelings, memories, and urges the conscious individual can tolerate and those it cannot

repression—a hypothetical, unconscious process by which unacceptable (often trauma-related) thoughts and feelings are kept out of conscious awareness

Several experts provide detailed information on psychodynamic therapy for PTSD.[61,121–123]

self-cohesion—knowledge and integration of previously unconscious motivations

In some ways, BPP's goals are similar to PE/CBT's, yet it has different conceptual underpinnings and therapeutic techniques.

exists only one randomized clinical trial on treatment efficacy for reducing PTSD symptoms.

Much more research is needed to demonstrate psychodynamic treatment efficacy for PTSD.

This study involved the use of BPP for 18 sessions and compared results with hypnotherapy and CBT (systematic desensitization). BPP effectively reduced PTSD intrusion and avoidance symptoms by approximately 40 percent. This improvement was:[125]

- ▶ Sustained for three months
- ▶ Comparable to results from the other two treatments
- ▶ Significantly greater than a wait-list group that received no treatment

Based on clinical case studies, rather than empirical research, it has been suggested that psychodynamic psychotherapy may be useful for patients with complex PTSD.[126–128]

Group Therapies

Group therapies utilize a psychodynamic focus, CBT focus, or supportive techniques (each with a different approach) and can be combined with the other therapies.[129] In all cases, trauma survivors learn about PTSD and help each other with the aid of a professional clinician.

Group therapy is generally well-accepted by those who have all survived the same type of trauma (e.g., war, rape, torture, terrorist bombing, etc.). As members share experiences, they become connected to one another by recognizing their common human fears, frailties, guilt, shame, and demoralization. Through clinician guidance, validation, and normalization of these thoughts, feelings, and behaviors, group members acquire more adaptive coping strategies, symptom reduction, and/or derivation of meaning from the traumatic experience.

Psychodynamic/Interpersonal Focus Group Therapy

Group members help one another understand how their assumptions about themselves (e.g., weak, shameful, guilty, undeserving) have been shaped and distorted by their prior experiences and traumatic encounters. By revisiting this material in the safety of the group, they are empowered to confront the traumatic memories to gain new insight about these memories and themselves, and to integrate such knowledge into their lives. Personal growth results from improved ego strength, insight, and self-understanding. Although symptom reduction is not the major treatment goal, therapists expect that resolution of trauma-related disruptions to normal psychic processes will promote PTSD amelioration.[130]

Interpersonal group therapy also emphasizes insight-based learning and change. Here the focus is on interpersonal, rather than intrapsychic factors that contribute to ongoing distress. Relationship difficulties are addressed in terms of relationship disputes, social deficits, role transitions, and relationship losses. The objective is to identify personal behaviors that discourage others from providing social support and/or that make them vulnerable to exploitation from others. This would include, of course, PTSD-related symptoms and behaviors that adversely affect interpersonal relationships.

Efficacy—All studies on psychodynamic or interpersonal group therapy have been conducted with female survivors of (childhood and/or adult) sexual trauma. Most studies have been small and have had varied results when compared to wait-list controls. In some cases better results were observed among group members, in comparison with wait-list controls; in others, there was no difference. In one study, it was found that positive outcomes are much less likely when one or more group members has borderline personality disorder. Findings from groups utilizing interpersonal therapy are generally stronger than from those applying psychodynamic techniques, although both group approaches were associated with small to medium positive pre-post changes.[131]

Cognitive-Behavioral Focus Group Therapy

These groups embody the concepts and approaches described earlier for individual cognitive-behavioral therapy (see pages 43–52).[87,129] One specific group approach uses both exposure and cognitive therapy; the clinician guides one group member at a time through a typical exposure session followed by cognitive restructuring.[132] During the exposure session, the other members are vicariously exposed to their own traumatic memories through observing someone else's treatment.

Group members do more for each other than provide social support. They validate one another's posttraumatic reactions, share their struggles to cope with PTSD-related problems, and provide honest criticism of fellow members' maladaptive coping behavior based on accurate empathy and their own experiences. Since group time is limited, group members must carry out homework assignments in which they focus or expose themselves to traumatic material. This homework is done through writing exercises or by repeatedly listening to an audiotape previously recorded during a group session in which they underwent exposure to their own traumatic material. An important challenge in CBT group therapy is to ensure that each group member has an adequate dose of exposure and cognitive restructuring. This can only be accomplished through out-of-session homework. Indeed, when comparing preliminary

> During the retelling of the trauma story, emotion is mobilized; as a result, it is hoped, the patient experiences a profound catharsis or "abreaction." Achieving catharsis and gaining insight is an important mediator of recovery in this treatment approach.
>
> The ultimate goal for both psychodynamic and cognitive-behavioral group therapy is for group members to gain "authority" over traumatic material so that it no longer is a dominant factor in their lives.[129]

> Other group approaches employing CBT have been utilized, most notably CPT (see pages 48–49) and SIT (see page 49).[86,89]

findings from a very successful CBT group for Vietnam veterans with PTSD[133] with a less successful study,[134] it appears that veterans in the successful group had an average of 22 exposures to traumatic material in contrast to only 10 exposures for the less successful group.

Efficacy—There have been few rigorous trials of cognitive-behavioral group treatments and results are mixed. There have been both positive and large negative focus group trials with Vietnam veterans with war-zone-related trauma and a positive trial with women with PTSD related to childhood sexual abuse. Assessment of adequate dosage for each group member of exposure and cognitive restructuring remains an important challenge. Group treatment with imagery rehearsal therapy has also had positive results, as mentioned previously. Seeking Safety, a widely used CBT group approach for people with co-occurring PTSD and substance abuse, has yet to demonstrate efficacy for either disorder, although it appears to be a very promising engagement strategy to get these complicated patients into treatment.

Supportive Group Therapy

Supportive groups emphasize here-and-now issues and try to redirect discussion of past traumatic experiences to present problems or concerns.

Supportive group therapy provides psychoeducation and focuses on members' current life issues.[129,130] The goal of treatment is not to revisit, reframe, or master traumatic material, but to discuss here-and-now issues. Traumatic consequences, as expressed by PTSD symptoms, are only relevant if they affect present-day functioning. To improve emotional and interpersonal comfort and overall functioning, group members are encouraged to develop better interpersonal and coping skills, problem-solving skills, and more adaptive responses to predictable challenges.

Efficacy—Results with supportive therapy have been mixed. In a recent large randomized trial in which 360 Vietnam combat veterans with PTSD were randomized to 30 weekly sessions of either CBT or supportive therapy, results were similar for both groups. Thirty-eight percent of the veterans improved, 43 percent were unchanged, and 18 percent had worse symptoms after treatment.[134]

One controlled trial of supportive group therapy for female sexual assault survivors showed a 19 to 30 percent reduction in intrusion and avoidance symptoms that was maintained for six months.[86]

In summary, there are relatively few well-designed randomized clinical trials of any specific group approach. At this time there is no conclusive evidence that one approach is superior to the other, although CBT group therapy has been studied most frequently and has the most empirical support. At this time, it appears that all group therapeutic approaches are superior to wait-list controls, but the strength of this evidence is modest, at best.

Couples/Family Therapy

This treatment focuses on how relationships either can be disrupted by a family member's PTSD (systemic treatment) or can foster a better healing environment for the PTSD patient (supportive treatment).[135–140] There have been a few trials of CBT approaches for families and couples.

Behavioral Family Therapy (BFT)[141] is a treatment that combines exposure therapy with BFT. Although the BFT group showed better problem-solving skills at the end of treatment, improvement in PTSD symptoms was no better than exposure alone.

Cognitive-Behavioral Couples Treatment (CBCT) addresses PTSD and relationship problems simultaneously. It had very promising results in an uncontrolled pilot study with male Vietnam veterans and their partners.[142,143]

Lifestyle Management Course, a one-week, 35-hour course, had promising results for 111 male veterans and their partners. Besides reductions in PTSD, both veterans and partners reported significant reductions in anxiety, depression, and stress.[144]

Although promising, all of these studies are limited by small samples, lack of a control group, and lack of replication. Given how much PTSD can disrupt marital and family life, it is hoped that research in this area will receive more attention in the near future.

Hypnosis

There have been only two randomized trials with hypnosis for PTSD patients. In an older study, hypnosis demonstrated equal efficacy with both CBT (systematic desensitization) and psychodynamic psychotherapy.[125,145] More recently, CBT plus hypnosis was compared with CBT alone. Both treatments were more effective than supportive counseling immediately after treatment and at 3-year follow-up. It also appeared that CBT plus hypnosis more effectively reduced intrusion symptoms than CBT alone.[146]

It is not clear what unique advantages hypnosis provides for PTSD treatment. It is now utilized primarily as an adjunctive procedure for confronting difficult traumatic memories, nightmares, or dissociative symptoms.[145]

There are currently no data supporting social rehabilitative therapies for PTSD. It is an important area for future research.

Social Rehabilitative Therapies

Effective for those with persistent mental illnesses (e.g., schizophrenia, severe affective disorders), these therapies are used with chronic, severe, and incapacitating PTSD (often indistinguishable from other persistent mental illness).[17,147] The seven psychosocial rehabilitation techniques recommended for severe and chronic PTSD are the following:[148]

1. Patient education services
2. Self-care/independent living skills techniques
3. Supported housing services
4. Family support
5. Social skills training
6. Supported employment techniques/sheltered workshops
7. Case management

What Psychosocial Treatments Are Available for Children and Adolescents with PTSD?

Treatments for children and adolescents are often age-appropriate interventions extrapolated from adult treatment methods. For children who develop PTSD, the impact of the trauma as well as the expression of symptoms may be significantly affected by the developmental stage at which the trauma occurred.[149,150] For example:

► Abused infants and toddlers may have impaired ability to form attachments with significant others.

► Traumatized preschoolers, who lack the conceptual and communication capacities of older individuals, may express nonverbal symptoms (e.g., aggression, withdrawal, or sleep problems).

► Trauma in children may result in restructured emotional expression, social isolation, problems with impulse control, self-injurious behaviors, dissociation, and development of *dissociative identity disorder* or borderline personality disorder.

► Trauma during adolescence may be expressed by anger, alienation, reckless behavior, and substance abuse. It may severely disrupt normal adult development by producing problems separating from parents, personality evolution, symbolic thinking, and moral development.[151–155]

dissociative identity disorder—previously called multiple personality disorder, which is characterized by one's personality becoming so fragmented that pronounced changes in behavior and reactivity are noticed between different social situations or social roles

CBT for Children and Adolescents

According to Cohen, Mannarino, and Deblinger,[156] all CBT approaches for children have common components that can be summarized by the acronym PRACTICE: Parental treatment component (including parenting skills); Psychoeducation; Relaxation and stress management skills; Affective expression and modulation skills; Cognitive coping skills, Trauma narrative and cognitive processing of the child's traumatic experiences; In-vivo desensitization to trauma reminders; Conjoint child-parent sessions; and Enhancing safety and future development.

Trauma-Focused CBT (TF-CBT) includes all of the PRACTICE components. In five randomized trials with over 500 children and adolescents exposed to sexual abuse, TF-CBT proved superior to comparison treatments for improving PTSD symptoms. It has also been effective for improving depression, social skills, sexual behavior, and parenting skills.[156]

Other promising CBT approaches include the following:

Cognitive-Based CBT (CBC) is designed for children exposed to single-incident trauma (such as motor vehicle accidents, interpersonal trauma, or witnessing violence). In a single trial, it was superior to wait list for reducing PTSD symptoms.[157]

Seeking Safety (mentioned previously, see page 56) has had promising results with children dually diagnosed with PTSD and substance use disorder.[158]

There are a number of other CBT approaches, currently in preliminary stages of testing, that hold promise for the future. A comprehensive review of these treatments can be found elsewhere.[156]

School-Based Treatments for Children and Adolescents

This category covers a variety of interventions including (a) schoolwide curricular interventions; (b) interventions designed for at-risk students; and (c) school-based treatments for students with trauma-related symptoms. Most interventions tested to date have focused on at-risk children, identified through some sort of screening protocol to determine a need for treatment. Most interventions utilized in schools are based on a CBT approach and incorporate the PRACTICE components mentioned previously. School-based approaches are generally delivered in a group, often in a classroom-style format rather than in an individual or conjoint child/parent format.[159]

Three treatments have been tested that all draw heavily on well-established CBT techniques. They focus on symptom reduction as well as developing coping skills (with respect to affect regulation and anxiety reduction). Each treatment includes specific techniques to focus on the traumatic event. All have proven effective for reducing trauma-related symptoms.

Cognitive-Behavioral Intervention for Trauma in Schools (CBITS)[160] has been used effectively with sixth and seventh graders and with recent immigrant students.

Multimodality Trauma Treatment (MMTT)[161] has significantly reduced PTSD, depression, and anxiety among elementary and junior high school students.

UCLA Trauma/Grief Program[162] has proven successful among school-age survivors of the earthquake in Armenia, in postwar Bosnia, and with children in Southern California. See Jaycox, Stein & Amaya-Jackson[159] for further details.

A consistent body of evidence supports the efficacy of CBT treatment for children with PTSD.

Psychodynamic Therapy for Child Trauma

Five randomized trials support the efficacy of psychodynamic approaches.

Child-Parent Psychotherapy (CPP) consists of 50 weekly sessions in which the goal is to strengthen the child-parent relationship. The therapist focuses on mothers' and children's maladaptive representations of themselves and each other, and on interactions and behaviors that interfere with the child's mental health.[163] During the treatment parent and child develop a joint narrative of the traumatic event and identify traumatic triggers that set off dysregulated and maladaptive behaviors. Three randomized trials with CPP have all been conducted with preschool children exposed to maltreatment and domestic violence.

Attachment and Biobehavioral Catch-Up (ABC)[164] was specifically developed for young maltreated children in foster care. The goal is to reduce children's affect dysregulation by improving the child-caregiver relationship. Children-caregiver dyads showed significant improvement in their relationships in comparison to a psychoeducational intervention.

It is worth noting that participants in the three CPP and one ABC trials were predominantly from ethnic minorities.

The fifth randomized psychodynamic treatment trial compared individual psychoanalytically based psychotherapy with a psychoeducation-based group treatment. Sexually abused girls aged 6–14 years who received individual psychotherapy exhibited significantly greater reductions in PTSD symptoms at 1 and 2 year follow-up assessments.[165]

Comparing the child versus adult treatment research on psychodynamic treatment, it is noteworthy that more randomized trials have been done with children than adults. As with adults, many of the outcomes concerned intrapsychic and interpersonal outcomes than specific reduction of PTSD symptoms.

Creative Arts Therapies for Children and Adults

Creative arts therapies have been utilized for many psychiatric disorders. These include art therapy, dance/movement therapy, psychodrama, music therapy, and poetry therapy. They have also been used for PTSD patients and have generated a great deal of enthusiasm among their practitioners.[166] Unfortunately, there is only one empirical trial of creative arts therapy. It involved 85 7- to 17-year-olds with traumatic injury who received one session of art therapy. There was no difference in overall PTSD symptom severity in comparison with the treatment-as-usual group; the art therapy group did exhibit a significant decrease in avoidance symptoms at one month that was sustained for one month.[167] Clearly, much more work in this area is needed.

Combined Treatments

As indicated previously, many CBT protocols include more than one modality. For example, a 10-session CBT treatment protocol may include psychoeducation, exposure, cognitive, and relaxation therapy. It is not uncommon for a person receiving a psychosocial treatment to also receive concurrent medication. We will review some of the research on combined psychotherapy and pharmacotherapy in Chapter 5.

Key Concepts for Chapter 4

1. Psychoeducation helps patients understand that their symptoms reflect a response to catastrophic stress shared by many as well as the nature of the disorder and its impact on their lives. It is especially useful as a societal and community intervention, using mass media, following terrorism or mass casualties due to a natural disaster.

2. Psychoeducational interventions help patients achieve normalization in their lives, remove self-blame and doubt, correct misunderstandings about what is causing their symptoms, and enhance the clinician's credibility as someone who truly understands the patient's struggles.

3. Individual psychotherapy used to treat PTSD includes cognitive behavioral treatments (CBT), eye movement desensitization (EMDR), and psychodynamic psychotherapy. Of these, research suggests that CBT and EMDR approaches are the most effective.

4. Prolonged exposure therapy (PE), which focuses on the details of the traumatic event itself, and cognitive therapy, which focuses on changing how the patient perceives the traumatic event, appear to be equally effective for improving PTSD symptoms (60–70 percent) when studied alone and in combination.

5. Despite questions regarding its mechanism of action, empirical evidence suggests that EMDR is effective in treating PTSD, perhaps as effective as CBT.

6. It is difficult to determine the effectiveness of psychodynamic treatment due to its focus on psychic processes instead of psychiatric symptoms, which are far more measurable.

7. Group therapies are often well-accepted by people who have survived the same type of trauma (e.g., veterans). These approaches use psychodynamic, CBT, or supportive techniques and can be combined with other therapies. Although there have been some positive results, there have been few rigorous trials, to date, to demonstrate the efficacy of group therapy.

8. Children and adolescents with PTSD face additional treatment challenges based on their development stage, when the trauma occurred, and the impact of that stage on how they were able to put what was happening into some overall context. Family

and school involvement appear critical to treatment success.

9. There is strong evidence that CBT approaches for children and adolescents, especially TF-CBT, are very effective.

10. School-based interventions for children and adolescents have proven to be effective.

Chapter 5
Pharmacological Treatments for PTSD

This chapter answers the following questions:

▶ **How Does the Human Stress Response Occur?**—This section details the neurobiology involved in the "fight, flight, or freeze" reaction as well as in the general adaptation syndrome.

▶ **What Psychobiological Abnormalities Occur in Those with PTSD?**—This section covers abnormalities in brain function and structure as well as alterations in the adrenergic, HPA, and serotonergic systems.

▶ **How Can Medications Best Be Used to Treat PTSD?**—This section discusses specific drugs available for PTSD treatment and their efficacy as well as treatment strategies.

MOST medical treatments for PTSD target abnormalities in the multiple biological systems involved with a person's response to stress. This section reviews:

1. Psychobiology of the body's general response to stress
2. Abnormalities in the human stress response associated with PTSD
3. Specific medication treatments that target these abnormalities
4. Corresponding efficacy research

How Does the Human Stress Response Occur?

Through evolution, humans have acquired a number of biological mechanisms for coping with the many different kinds of stressors normally encountered in the course of a lifetime. The most important brain structures involved in the stress response are the amygdala, hippocampus, and prefrontal cortex.

The *amygdala* is the part of the brain that processes emotional input, especially the fear, helplessness, and horror associated with exposure to a traumatic event. It is the ignition switch and plays a key role in coordinating the response to threat or stress. It mobilizes a number of cortical and subcortical brain mechanisms, initially through activation of corticotropin-releasing factor (CRF). CRF activates two major components of the human stress response—the "fight, flight, or freeze" reaction and the general adaptation syndrome.

amygdala—principal nucleus in the brain for appraising emotional input and threatening stimuli and then mobilizing protective, defensive, or escape behavior

The hippocampus plays a major role in learning and memory and is involved in converting short-term to long-term memory. It provides a mental map or context for remembering traumatic events.

The medial prefrontal cortex (mPFC) regulates emotion and arousal. It is the major brain structure that can exert restraint on the amygdala.

Fight, Flight, or Freeze Reaction

sympathetic nervous system—part of the autonomic nervous system that regulates arousal functions such as heart rate and blood flow

This reaction refers to the amydala's mobilization of the *sympathetic nervous system* (SNS). SNS mechanisms are activated in response to a threat.[168] During this reaction, the heart pumps more blood to the muscles, which enables them to perform defensive ("fight"), escape ("flight"), or hiding ("freeze") movements necessary for survival. This reaction begins in the brain via a complex array of neurobiological mechanisms that have evolved to detect danger, to experience fear, and to set off a sequence of adaptive, defensive, escape, and hiding responses.

neurotransmitters—chemical messengers that transmit signals from one nerve cell to another to elicit physiological responses

Several important brain and SNS chemicals (*neurotransmitters*) that relay signals from one neuron to the next mediate the fight, flight, or freeze response, called an *adrenergic response* because norepinephrine and epinephrine are also called noradrenaline and adrenaline. Adrenergic agents augment or attenuate such responses in the brain, heart, blood vessels, and elsewhere.

adrenergic response—neuronal activation mediated by either norepinephrine (noradrenaline) or epinephrine (adrenaline)

Although the fight, flight, or freeze response was described more than 80 years ago with regard to the SNS and muscle activity, we have only recently come to understand how the amygdala, hippocampus, mPFC, and other brain structures react to threat and activate other neurobiological responses. When faced with a dangerous or stressful situation, the amygdala releases CRF, which activates the neurons in the locus coeruleus—a small cluster of nerve cells that contains most of the brain's adrenergic neurons. Locus coeruleus neurons activate brain centers (such as the hypothalamus, hippocampus, and cerebral cortex) that mediate arousal, emotional reactivity, and memory as well as the SNS, which instigates the fight, flight, or freeze response.[169,170] This same hormone (CRF) activates an additional response to stress—the general adaptation syndrome.

See page 71 for an explanation of how neurotransmitters function.

The General Adaptation Syndrome

hypothalamic-pituitary-adrenocortical (HPA) axis—three anatomic structures that participate collectively in the hormonal response to stress: the hypothalamus (in the brain), the pituitary gland, and the outer layer (cortex) of the adrenal gland

The general adaptation syndrome involves the second major system that responds to stress.[171] It is a hormonal rather than a neurotransmitter response and focuses on the *hypothalamic-pituitary-adrenocortical (HPA) axis*.

The hypothalamus—a small, midline nucleus on the underside of the brain—releases CRF into the bloodstream, which carries it rapidly to the nearby pituitary gland, provoking the release of adrenocorticotropic hormone (ACTH). ACTH is then carried by the bloodstream to the adrenal gland (perched atop the kidney), which releases *cortisol*. Cortisol has been called the "stress hormone" because blood cortisol levels are elevated during the normal human response to stress.

Many other neurobiological systems also participate in the human stress response, including the immunological system, the thyroid system, and other neurotransmitter and hormonal systems.[169,170,172]

The neurotransmitter serotonin is intimately involved in both adrenergic and HPA activity. It also facilitates inhibition of amygdala activity. Primarily located in the brainstem raphe nuclei, which have abundant reciprocal interactions with the adrenergic and many other brain neurotransmitter HPA systems, serotonin can facilitate the human stress response.[170] The diagram in Figure 5.1 on page 68 depicts major brain areas involved in this response.

The following discussion reviews abnormalities that result from trauma. On the horizon, research on medications that normalize the unique pathophysiology of PTSD appears to promise more effective medications in the future. Such medications will most probably not be traditional antidepressants or anxiolytics, but pharmacological agents that act on CRF—a key component of the human stress response. CRF antagonists are new medications, undergoing preliminary testing, which, potentially, might moderate the entire human stress response. Neuropeptide Y enhancers, that antagonize CRF actions, might be another class of medications to test, as well as other neuropeptides that affect these mechanisms.[15]

Since the systems affected by PTSD are key psychobiological mechanisms, advances in our basic understanding of human learning, memory, coping, and adaptation will accompany progress in this field.

What Psychobiological Abnormalities Occur in Those with PTSD?

In the normal stress response, the amygdala becomes acutely activated in reaction to threat. It mobilizes adrenergic, HPA and other stress-induced activity. Later, when the danger has passed, the amygdala returns to its normal baseline functioning, probably due, in part, to mPFC restraint. Our current model of PTSD, however, is a stress response that doesn't know when to

cortisol—a hormone that increases energy by raising blood glucose levels, decreases immune processes, and causes other metabolic and neurobiological actions

Medications that enhance serotonergic activity are classified as selective serotonin reuptake inhibitors (SSRIs), some of which have proven effective in PTSD treatment.

Figure 5.1   Human Stress Response

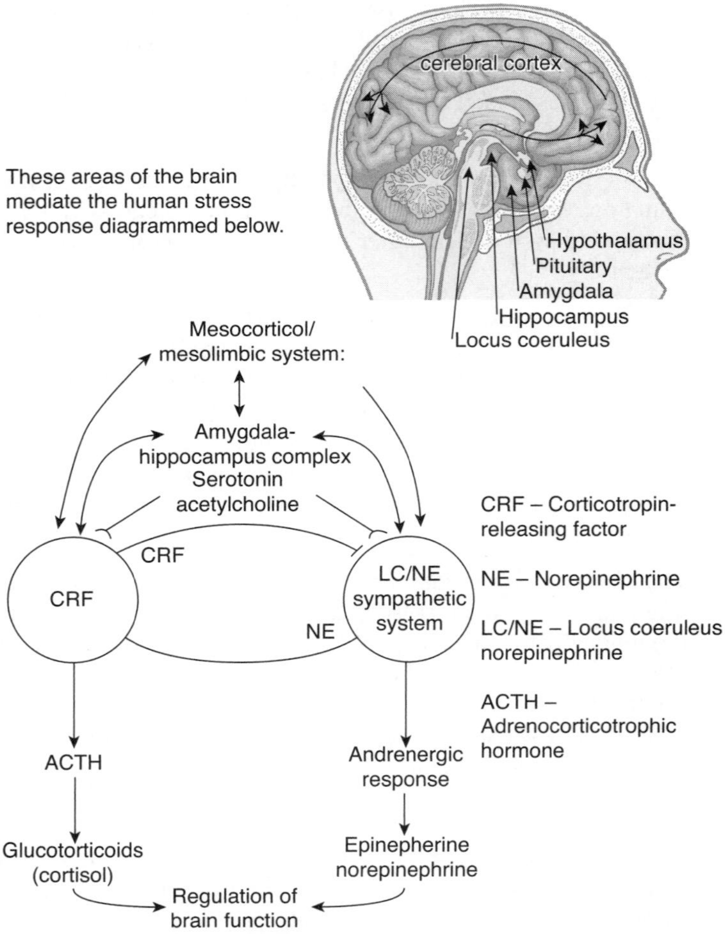

These areas of the brain mediate the human stress response diagrammed below.

Source: Diagram adapted from and reprinted with permission of Chrousos & Gold (1992).[172]

quit. It is like a perfect storm in which the amygdala remains in a state of excessive arousal while the mPFC is unable to exercise its usual restraint. This model predicts that any medication that either reduces amygdala activity or increases mPFC activity would be expected to be effective for treating PTSD.

The psychobiology of PTSD is complicated. Research indicates that other PTSD-related psychobiological abnormalities involve

Figure 5.2 Key Brain Structures in Fear Conditioning and PTSD

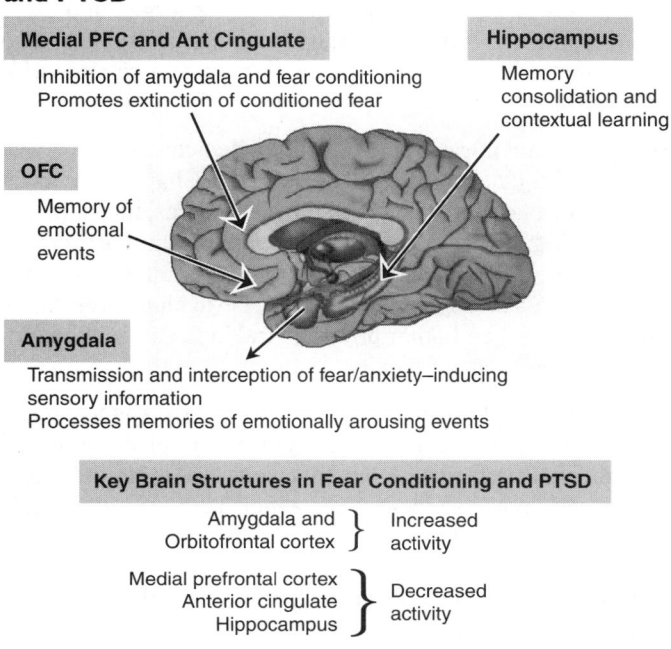

Medial PFC and Ant Cingulate

Inhibition of amygdala and fear conditioning
Promotes extinction of conditioned fear

Hippocampus

Memory consolidation and contextual learning

OFC

Memory of emotional events

Amygdala

Transmission and interception of fear/anxiety–inducing sensory information
Processes memories of emotionally arousing events

Key Brain Structures in Fear Conditioning and PTSD

Amygdala and Orbitofrontal cortex } Increased activity

Medial prefrontal cortex
Anterior cingulate
Hippocampus } Decreased activity

thyroid, opioid, immunological, and other neurotransmitter, neuropeptide, or neurohormonal systems.[15] This chapter focuses only on the major PTSD-altered systems on which currently utilized pharmacological agents have the most influence. As we learn more about different brain mechanisms that PTSD affects, new medications will evolve to act on systems other than the adrenergic and serotonergic. Indeed, some medications, traditionally used to treat seizure disorders (e.g., antiepileptic drugs), have also been tested in PTSD. These medications exert their actions on the glutamatergic and GABA systems, which are the brain's major excitatory and inhibitory systems, respectively (see below). More detailed information on the psychobiology of the human stress response can be found elsewhere.[169,170]

Research indicates that the adrenergic HPA and serotonergic systems as well as CRF function abnormally in people with PTSD.

psychological probe—a visual or auditory stimulus reminiscent of a traumatic experience to which a person with PTSD is exposed

pharmacological probe—a drug that can activate psychobiological mechanisms involved in the stress response

The prefrontal cortex is the part of the brain that exerts the major restraining influence on the amygdala.

Adrenergic System

For those with PTSD, it appears that the adrenergic (and SNS) system is much more active than in normal individuals. The most dramatic illustrations of this finding are experiments with *psychological* and *pharmacological probes.*

A typical psychological probe for a motor vehicle accident survivor with PTSD (such as Mary T. described in Chapter 2) may be the sound of a large truck or the squeal of brakes, the sight of a truck crashing into a car, or someone reciting details of a similar accident.[173,174] Under such conditions, Mary T. would experience excessive SNS activation exhibited by a rise in blood pressure, a racing heart rate, and other physiological indications of heightened SNS physiological activity.

Such physiological abnormalities can also cause abnormal elevations of blood or urinary norepinephrine as well as increased activation of the amygdala, locus coeruleus, and other brain centers. Mary T. may also experience abnormalities in the brain's normal blood flow; these include increased blood flow to the amygdala and reduced circulation to the mPFC and hippocampus. Motor vehicle accident survivors who do not develop PTSD do not exhibit this heightened reactivity of adrenergic mechanisms in the SNS and brain.

A typical pharmacological probe is yohimbine, which causes excessive firing of adrenergic neurons.[175] Research with yohimbine has shown that the adrenergic system is abnormally sensitive in PTSD. Indeed, giving an intravenous dose of yohimbine to

From the Patient's Perspective

I've been on the medication for three weeks now. I really didn't want to take it, but Dr. Owen convinced me that it might help me function better. It's really getting a lot easier to get behind the wheel of the car. I still don't like the trucks, but at least I can deal with them now. Therapy is really helpful. I can handle the memories a lot better and have begun to discover things that happened after the crash that I had completely forgotten. It's also easier to concentrate, and I can sit at the computer for a few hours. Dr. Owen wants me to consider easing back to work on a part-time basis. I don't think I'm ready, but I'll give it a try if she thinks I should.

Mary T. might provoke a panic attack or even a flashback of the truck crashing into her car. Yohimbine does not produce such a response in people without PTSD. Yohimbine can even affect blood flow in the brain, thereby demonstrating the abnormal adrenergic sensitivity of those with PTSD.[175]

HPA System

People with PTSD have shown a variety of HPA abnormalities, including elevated cerebrospinal CRF levels and abnormal serum and urinary cortisol levels (although study results are mixed).[176]

Although there is general agreement that those with PTSD have a significantly altered HPA system, there are a number of scientific controversies regarding the precise nature of HPA abnormalities. There is also evidence that people who develop PTSD have vulnerable HPA systems and that the traumatic event unmasked a biological abnormality that impairs their capacity to cope with catastrophic stress.[177]

Serotonergic System

Research on the serotonergic system in PTSD is at a much more preliminary stage than research on adrenergic or HPA mechanisms. It appears, however, that serotonin plays an important modulatory role in both systems and is a key component of the human stress response.[170] Clinical studies show abnormalities in serotonergic mechanisms in PTSD patients.

Neurotransmission

Medications used to treat PTSD modify neurotransmission in serotonergic and adrenergic neurons. Neurons communicate by releasing neurotransmitters into the *synaptic cleft*. The *presynaptic neuron* produces, packages, releases, and delivers the neurotransmitter into the synapse, where it can diffuse across to the *postsynaptic neuron*.

Neurotransmitters attach to a specific postsynaptic *receptor*. The neurotransmitter forms a temporary binding complex with the receptor, analogous to a "lock-and-key" formation.

Binding of the neurotransmitter to the receptor results in a chemical change that leads to a biological response, such as a behavior, thought, or reaction.

After their presynaptic release, most neurotransmitters are subsequently reabsorbed by a specialized reuptake site located on the presynaptic neuron. The reuptake mechanism is selective for serotonin or norepinephrine, respectively. Various

synaptic cleft—the space between one neuron and the next that must be traversed by neurotransmitters

presynaptic neuron—the neuron that initiates neurotransmission by releasing the neurotransmitter into the synaptic cleft

postsynaptic neuron—the downstream neuron that is the target of neurotransmission

receptors—membrane-bound protein molecules with a highly specific shape that facilitate binding by neurotransmitters or medications

medications affect different parts of the neurotransmitter system. These include:

- ▶ Selective serotonin reuptake inhibitors (SSRIs)
- ▶ Tricyclic antidepressants (TCAs)
- ▶ Venlafaxine
- ▶ Monoamine oxidase inhibitors (MAOIs)

Figure 5.3 illustrates what these medications block and the results. For more detailed information on these and other medications used to treat PTSD, review the following section.

Figure 5.3　Medication Impacts

Medications	What They Block	What's the Result
SSRIs	Presynaptic reuptake site on serotonergic neurons	More serotonin available to bind postsynaptic receptors
TCAs Venlafaxine	Presynaptic reuptake of both serotonin and norepinephrine	More serotonin and norepinephrine available to bind to postsynaptic receptors
MAOIs	Inhibits enzyme MAO, which destroys serotonin and norepinephrine	More serotonin and norepinephrine available for presynaptic release

Source: Adapted from Friedman MJ (2003). Pharmacological management of PTSD, *Primary Psychiatry* 10, 66–73.

How Can Medications Best Be Used to Treat PTSD?

In view of the great success of cognitive-behavioral therapy (CBT), pharmacotherapy is only one of several treatment options for PTSD patients.[73] Medication may be a good choice when:[41]

- ▶ Patient acceptability of such an approach is high.
- ▶ Comorbid conditions are present that are responsive to pharmacotherapy (e.g., depression, panic disorder, social phobia, and obsessive-compulsive disorder).
- ▶ CBT treatment is unavailable.

Figure 5.4, on pages 74–75, summarizes the current clinical literature on pharmacological trials. (More comprehensive reviews can be found elsewhere.)[178,179] It provides information on medication class, specific medication, therapeutic dose range, clinical indications, and contraindications. Of these medications, only two SSRIs are approved by the FDA for the treatment of PTSD

The Handbook of PTSD: Science and Practice *includes a chapter titled "Pharmacotherapy for PTSD" that offers a comprehensive review of PTSD pharmacology.*[178]

Chapter 4 provides detailed information on CBT treatment for those with PTSD.

Laboratory research indicates a strong rationale for considering antiadrenergic agents; however, there will need to be more extensive testing to establish these agents' usefulness for PTSD patients.

(paroxetine and sertraline). SSRIs are considered the first-line treatment for PTSD because they:[180–183]

▶ Have broad-spectrum effects against all PTSD symptom clusters

▶ Are effective against many comorbid disorders

▶ Are effective against associated symptoms, such as impulsivity, aggression, and suicidal thoughts

Venlafaxine, which produces presynaptic blockade of both serotonin (like an SSRI) and norepinephrine, is also a first-line treatment for PTSD.[184,185]

Atypical antipsychotics may effectively augment first- or second-line medication treatment; however, much more research is needed.

Second-line medications include mirtazapine, prazosin, MAOIs, and TCAs. Evidence favoring the use of these agents is not as compelling as evidence for using SSRIs or venlafaxine.[178,179]

Other medications in Figure 5.4 include antiadrenergic agents and atypical antipsychotics. Laboratory research indicates a strong rationale for considering antiadrenergic agents; however, only prazosin has been shown to be effective so far, and there remain questions about whether this effectiveness is limited to reduction of traumatic nightmares and improvement of insomnia, or whether it is effective against all PTSD symptoms. There will need to be more extensive testing to establish the usefulness of other antiadrenergic agents for PTSD patients.[178,179]

Atypical antipsychotics have been shown to be effective for adjunctive therapy. Although they have demonstrated little efficacy on their own, when combined with first- or second-line medications, they have demonstrated effectiveness in randomized trials.[178,179]

D-cycloserine (DCS) is a unique medication that potentiates glutamate at n-methyl-d-aspartate (NMDA) receptors, which are critical in learning new behaviors. Since animal research had shown that DCS accelerates extinction of fear conditioning, and since extinction is really learning a new response to a traumatic reminder, DCS has been combined with exposure therapy (which promotes extinction of fear-conditioned PTSD symptoms). In practice, DCS is given before each session of exposure therapy. Preliminary research indicates that that clinical improvement takes place more quickly when DCS is combined with exposure therapy than when exposure therapy is provided without the medication. This raises the very exciting possibility that utilization of DCS may reduce the number of sessions of exposure therapy needed to achieve clinical success.[186,187] It should also be noted that in much of the current research DCS is combined with exposure therapy that is delivered in a virtual reality format. Finally, it must be stated that DCS is ineffective by itself; it is only useful when combined with exposure therapy.

Figure 5.4   Medications for PTSD—Indications and Contraindications*

Class**	Medication	Daily Dose Range (mg)	Indications	Contraindications
Selective Serotonin Reuptake Inhibitors (SSRIs)	Paroxetine*** Sertraline*** Fluoxetine Citalopram Fluvoxamine	10–60 50–200 20–80 20–60 50–300	• Reduce B, C, and D symptoms • Produce clinical global improvement • Effective treatment for depression, panic disorder, social phobia, and obsessive-compulsive disorder • Reduce associated symptoms (rage, aggression, impulsivity, suicidal thoughts)	• May produce insomnia, restlessness, nausea, decreased appetite, daytime sedation, nervousness, and anxiety • May produce sexual dysfunction, decreased libido, delayed orgasm, or anorgasmia • Clinically significant interactions with MAOIs • Significant interactions with hepatic enzymes produce other drug interactions • Concern about increased suicidal risk in children and adolescents
Other 2nd-Generation Antidepressants	Venlafaxine Mirtazapine Buproprion Trazadone	75–225 15–45 200–450 150–600	• Multisite trials indicate Venlafaxine is as effective as SSRIs • Effective for PTSD • Effectiveness in PTSD not established • (Trazadone) Limited efficacy by itself but is synergistic with SSRIs and may reduce SSRI-induced insomnia • All of these medications are useful in depression	• May exacerbate hypertension • May produce somnolence, increased appetite and weight gain • May exacerbate seizure disorder • May be too sedating, rare priapism; however, may be useful as a bedtime medication for SSRI-induced insomnia
Monoamine Oxidase Inhibitors (MAOIs)	Phenelzine	15–90	• Reduces B symptoms • Produces global improvement • Effective agent for depression, panic, and social phobia	• Risk of hypertensive crisis requires a strict dietary regimen • Contraindicated in combination with most other antidepressants, CNS stimulants, and decongestants • Contraindicated in patients with alcohol/substance abuse/dependency • May produce insomnia, hypotension, anticholinergic side effects, and severe liver toxicity

*Modified from Friedman & Davidson.[178]

**Anticonvulsants not shown because none has demonstrated efficacy for PTSD

***FDA approval as indicated treatment for PTSD

(*continued*)

Figure 5.4 (*Continued*)

Tricyclic Antidepressants (TCAs)	Imipramine	150–300	• Imipramine and Amitriptyline reduce B symptoms and produce global improvement • Effective antidepressant and antipanic agents • (Desipramine) Ineffective in one randomized clinical trial	• Anticholinergic side effects (dry mouth, rapid pulse, blurred vision, constipation) • May produce ventricular arrhythmias • May produce orthostatic hypotension, sedation, or arousal
	Amitriptyline	150–300		
	Desipramine	100–300		
Antiadrenergic Agents	Prazosin	6–10	• None of these medications have established efficacy in PTSD • Prazosin shown to have marked efficacy for PTSD nightmares and insomnia	• May produce hypotension or brachycardia • Use cautiously with hypotensive patients; titrate prazosin starting at 1 mg at bedtime and monitor blood pressure • Propranolol may produce depressive symptoms, psychomotor slowing, or bronchospasm
	Propranolol	40–160		
	Clonidine	0.2–0.6		
	Guanfacine	1–3		
Atypical Antipsychotics	Risperidone	4–16	• Effective role as augmenting agents with SSRIs and other treatments • Useful with aggressive patients	• Weight gain • (Olanzapine) Risk of type II diabetes
	Olanzapine	5–20		
	Quetiapine	50–750		

B Symptoms: intrusive recollections

C Symptoms: avoidant/numbing

D Symptoms: hyperarousal

Medications specifically not recommended for PTSD treatment include:

▶ Bupropion—No systematic testing in clinical trials.

▶ Carbamazepine, Valproate, and Other Anticonvulsants— A number of randomized trials with anticonvulsants have been very disappointing. They have not exhibited effectiveness in PTSD. More research is warranted, since there are theoretical reasons for thinking that these agents should be effective.

▶ Benzodiazepines—Appear ineffective against core PTSD symptoms and are potentially addictive.

▶ Conventional Antipsychotics—Poor side-effect profile compared to other agents, plus ineffective in practice.

▶ Nefazadone—This is an effective agent that has been removed by its manufacturer from the U.S. market because of liver toxicity (although generic nefazadone is available in the U.S.).[178,179]

SSRIs have proven effective against other major DSM-IV psychiatric disorders that are frequently comorbid with PTSD, such as depression, panic disorder, social phobia, and obsessive-compulsive disorder.

More recent findings indicate increased suicidal risk in children and adolescents taking SSRIs for depression.[190] Comparable research for this age group is lacking among PTSD patients. However, given these findings, suicidal risk should be carefully monitored at all times. The FDA has recently issued a very strong warning concerning SSRI use for children and adolescents.[191]

The following discussion reviews medications that are considered first- and second-line agents in more detail.

Selective Serotonin Reuptake Inhibitors (SSRIs)

Two SSRIs, sertraline and paroxetine, have received FDA approval based on positive findings in large, 12-week, multisite trials.[180–183] Improvement was found in 40 to 85 percent of respondents across trials. These agents offer many benefits, as shown in Figure 5.4.

Sertraline and paroxetine are broad-spectrum medications, which ameliorate symptoms from all three PTSD symptom clusters (e.g., reexperiencing, avoidant/numbing, and hyperarousal).

SSRIs also appear to reduce clinically significant symptoms often associated with PTSD, such as suicidal, aggressive, and impulsive behavior. Finally, as with all SSRIs, sertraline and paroxetine have a side-effect profile that is relatively benign compared to that of other medications. A large multisite trial and smaller open trials with fluoxetine indicate that this SSRI is also a very effective PTSD medication.[188] Although the SSRIs citalopram, escitalopram, and flovoxmine have not been studied sufficiently to warrant a recommendation, there have been promising findings with these agents.[178,179,189]

Despite SSRIs' clinical advantages and relatively low side-effect profile (compared to other antidepressant agents such as MAOIs and TCAs), they are poorly tolerated by some patients. Sexual dysfunction, agitation, and insomnia produced by SSRIs, especially fluoxetine, may be especially disruptive to PTSD patients. In addition, clinicians should exercise caution when prescribing SSRIs to patients taking other medications (especially MAOIs) due to serious drug interactions and SSRI-induced disruption of normal drug metabolism in the liver. Patients with gastrointestinal disorders, especially irritable bowel syndrome, sometimes experience problems when taking SSRIs because of increased intestinal motility. Finally, SSRIs have strong interactions with many other drugs, a factor that is important to keep in mind.

For patients who exhibit a partial response to SSRIs, one should consider continuation or augmentation strategies.[41] A nine-month trial with sertraline showed that approximately half of all patients failing to exhibit a successful clinical response after 12 weeks did respond when SSRI treatment continued for another 24 weeks.[192] Practically speaking, clinicians and patients usually are reluctant to stick with an ineffective medication for 36 weeks, as in this experiment, making augmentation strategies more appealing.

Two augmentation strategies have been tested when patients receiving SSRIs have only had a partial response to treatment. One is adding an atypical antipsychotic medication (see below). The other is keeping them on the medication but adding exposure therapy. There is one randomized trial in which partial responders to sertraline achieved complete remission after adding PE to their treatment.[193]

Augmentation Strategies

The following suggestions are not based on empirical evidence but on the author's clinical experience.

- ► Excessively aroused, hyperreactive, or dissociating patients might benefit from augmentation with an antiadrenergic agent (such as clonidine or guanfacine).
- ► Labile, impulsive, and/or aggressive patients might benefit from augmentation with an anticonvulsant.
- ► Fearful, hypervigilant, paranoid, and psychotic patients might benefit from an atypical antipsychotic.

Other Second-Generation Antidepressants

Venlafaxine, a powerful antidepressant that blocks presynaptic uptake of both serotonin and norepinephrine, appears to be very effective for PTSD, based on large, multisite trials.[184,185]

Mirtazapine has also proven effective in randomized trials.

Another second-generation antidepressant, buproprion, is not recommended for PTSD treatment due to insufficient efficacy data. Finally, as stated previously, nefazadone, an effective agent, is not recommended because of liver toxicity.

Since PTSD is often comorbid with major depression, many clinicians prefer to prescribe second-generation antidepressants because they are effective antidepressants with relatively benign side-effect profiles. It is important to recognize that effectiveness in depression does not automatically indicate effectiveness in PTSD. Indeed, some older antidepressants, MAOIs and TCAs, have proven effective for PTSD treatment, whereas bupropion has not.[178,179]

Monoamine Oxidase Inhibitors (MAOIs)

Comprehensive reviews of published findings on MAOI treatment indicate that MAOIs have produced moderate to good improvement in 82 percent of all patients, primarily due to reduction in reexperiencing symptoms, such as intrusive recollections, traumatic nightmares, and PTSD flashbacks.[194,195] Insomnia also improved; however, avoidant/numbing or hyperarousal symptoms of PTSD did not.

Although tested infrequently and not for almost 20 years, MAOIs have been very effective in most reported medication trials. Since they are also excellent antidepressants and antipanic agents, further research is definitely warranted.

A minimum of eight weeks of treatment with MAOIs or TCAs is necessary to achieve positive clinical results in veterans of military combat.

MAOI use has traditionally been limited when there are legitimate concerns of patients ingesting alcohol or pharmacologically contraindicated illicit drugs or not adhering to necessary dietary restrictions—resulting in severe and abrupt elevation of blood pressure (a hypertensive medical emergency). Testing with a much safer MAOI, moclobemide, suggests that this may prove to be an effective drug for PTSD in the future.

Tricyclic Antidepressants (TCAs)

Although TCAs are effective agents, side effects and failure to reduce avoidant/numbing symptoms have led to their replacement by SSRIs as first-line drugs in PTSD treatment.[178,179]

In an analysis of all published findings on TCA treatment for PTSD, 45 percent of patients showed moderate to good global improvement following treatment, in contrast to MAOIs, which produced global improvement in 82 percent of patients who received them.[195] As with MAOIs, most improvement was due to reductions in reexperiencing rather than avoidant/numbing or arousal symptoms. Furthermore, TCAs' anticholinergic, hypotensive, sedating, and cardiac arrhythmic side effects are poorly tolerated by many PTSD patients.

Antiadrenergic Agents

One of the earliest and most established findings in PTSD research is the excessive adrenergic reactivity among patients with the disorder.[170] Despite this robust, experimental finding and open trials dating back to 1984, antiadrenergic medications have been largely neglected until recently.[178,179]

The agents listed for this category in Figure 5.4 (pages 74–75) are safe medications used for many years in treating cardiovascular disease, especially hypertension and cardiac arrhythmias. Although all agents listed achieve the result—reduced adrenergic activity—three different mechanisms of action account for this:

- ▶ Prazosin—A postsynaptic, alpha-1 receptor antagonist
- ▶ Propranolol—A postsynaptic, beta adrenergic antagonist
- ▶ Clonidine and guanfacine—Presynaptic, alpha-2 receptor agonists, which reduce the amount of norepinephrine released into the synaptic cleft

The best research on this class of agents, well-controlled clinical trials, have focused on the alpha-1 postsynaptic antagonist, prazosin, which produced marked reduction in traumatic nightmares and improved sleep. Results regarding PTSD, however, have been mixed, indicating global improvement in overall PTSD symptom severity among veterans in one study but not another.[196,197] A large-scale trial with prazosin is currently in progress.

Propranolol was tested in sexually/physically abused children with chronic PTSD. It significantly reduced (by 25–64 percent) reexperiencing and arousal symptoms.[198] Unfortunately, this trial has not been repeated. Propranolol has also received attention as a prophylactic agent, which, when administered within hours of the traumatic event, might prevent the later development of PTSD. Results are inconclusive at this time (see Chapter 6).

Two randomized trials with the alpha-2 receptor agonist guanfacine have been negative despite laboratory evidence suggesting its potential effectiveness.[199,200] Clonidine, which has also been used successfully with Southeast Asian refugees with PTSD, has not been tested in a rigorous clinical trial. Therefore, neither of these agents can be recommended at this time.[201]

Anticonvulsants

Researchers hypothesize that following exposure to traumatic events, certain nuclei in the brain become "kindled" or "sensitized"; thereafter, they exhibit excessive responsivity to less intense, trauma-related stimuli.[202] Consistent with such a theory, there have been promising preliminary results. In five studies, carbamazepine produced reductions in 50–75 percent reexperiencing and arousal symptoms, while in three studies, valproate produced reductions in 60–75 percent avoidant/numbing and 50–65 percent arousal (but not reexperiencing) symptoms.[178,179] Unfortunately, three large-scale randomized trials with three agents, valproate, topirimate, and tiagabine, have indicated that these medications are no better than placebo.[203–205] Besides their lack of proven efficacy at this time, these drugs have a clinically significant spectrum of neurological, *hematopoietic,* gastrointestinal, and *teratogenic* side effects that may seriously complicate treatment. Since valproate's teratogenic effects occur early in the first trimester of pregnancy, it is best to use extreme caution with women of childbearing age.

Benzodiazepines

Clinicians often prescribe *benzodiazepines* for PTSD because of their proven efficacy as *anxiolytics.* This is unfortunate because studies with alprazolam and clonazepam indicate that these agents have no proven efficacy against core PTSD symptoms, whereas many more effective nonbenzodiazepine agents are available, as reviewed previously.[178,179,206] If prescribed, benzodiazepines typically improve sleep and reduce general anxiety, but have no salutary impact on the PTSD syndrome itself. Furthermore, there are potential risks of prescribing these agents, because they may be problematic for patients with past or present alcohol/drug misuse. In addition, alprazolam may

There is obviously a great need for more research with these anticonvulsant/antikindling agents to clarify their usefulness in PTSD treatment.

hematopoietic—suppression of the bone marrow's capacity to produce red and white blood cells

teratogenic—producing fetal abnormalities during pregnancy

benzodiazepine family of drugs—a very effective and widely prescribed class of medications for anxiety that includes diazepam, lorazepam, alprazolam, and clonazepam

anxiolytics—medications that relieve anxiety

produce rebound anxiety, which is poorly tolerated by PTSD patients. Since animal studies have shown that benzodiazepines interfere with extinction of fear conditioning, there is theoretical concern (and some clinical evidence) that benzodiazepines might interfere with prolonged exposure therapy.[207,208]

Antipsychotic Agents

Conventional antipsychotics are not recommended for PTSD patients, partly because more effective treatments are available and because *extrapyramidal* side effects make these agents a poor choice for PTSD treatment.[178,179]

extrapyramidal—uncontrollable involuntary motor movements or excessive rigidity

Atypical antipsychotics, especially risperidone and olanzapine, have proven to be effective adjunctive agents for patients who fail to achieve remission from monotherapy with a first-line medication. Several randomized trials have shown that when a patient receiving a medication (such as an SSRI) exhibits a partial or poor response after several months of treatment, his or her clinical response may be markedly improved when an atypical antipsychotic is added to the medication regimen. Therefore, atypical agents may have a unique niche as augmentation treatment for partial responders to SSRIs or other first- or second-line agents, especially for patients with intense hypervigilance/paranoia, agitation, dissociation, or brief psychotic reactions associated with their PTSD.[209–214]

Many Vietnam veterans in the 1970s received conventional antipsychotic agents to ameliorate intense PTSD-related hyperarousal, hypervigilance, dissociative symptoms, aggressivity, and reexperiencing symptoms. However, we now understand that PTSD is pathophysiologically different from psychotic disorders.

Although atypical antipsychotics have a more benign side effect profile than more conventional antipsychotic agents (especially with respect to tardive dyskinesia and other involuntary motor problems), there is concern that they may produce adverse effects leading to obesity, type-2 diabetes, and metabolic syndrome.

There are currently no approved or indicated medication treatments for children or adolescents with PTSD. Broad-spectrum agents such as SSRIs are probably a reasonable choice if pharmacotherapy is indicated (although suicidal thoughts and behavior must be monitored). Comorbid problems must also be taken into consideration such as depression, aggressive behavior, and attention deficit/hyperactivity disorder (ADHD).

Key Concepts for Chapter 5

1. Humans respond to stress using biological coping mechanisms instigated by the amygdala, which prompts release of corticotropin-releasing factor (CRF) which then promotes release of norepinephrine and cortisol. These mechanisms involve the sympathetic and central nervous systems' adrenergic neurotransmitters and the hypothalamic-pituitary-adrenocortical axis as well as the immunological, thyroid, and other neurotransmitter and hormonal systems.

2. SSRIs and venlafaxine represent the recommended first-line approach to treating PTSD based on large multi-site randomized clinical trials.

3. Second-line medications include mirtazapine, TCAs, and MAOIs, as well as prazosin for traumatic nightmares.

4. Atypical antipsychotic agents have proven effective as adjunctive agents to augment the efficacy of first- or second-line treatments. Augmentation with prolonged exposure therapy has also shown effectiveness in improving outcomes from patients who only achieved partial improvement during SSRI treatment.

5. D-cycloserine has shown great promise in augmenting prolonged exposure therapy and accelerating the rate of improvement.

6. Pharmacotherapy is the most reasonable approach to PTSD treatment when patients are in favor of taking medications, when comorbid conditions will also be addressed by the medications, and when CBT treatment is unavailable.

7. Benzodiazepines and anticonvulsant agents are not recommended for treating PTSD. They have not demonstrated efficacy in clinical trials and their side effects may cause adverse complications.

Chapter 6
Strategies for Acute Stress Reactions and Acute Stress Disorder (ASD)

This chapter answers the following questions:

▶ **What Are Normal Acute, Posttraumatic Distress Reactions?**—This section defines the four types of normal reactions people have to traumatic events.

▶ **What Treatment Approaches Are Used for Traumatic Event Survivors?**—This section defines the best psychological treatments that should be used during the immediate aftermath of a traumatic event.

▶ **What Is Acute Stress Disorder (ASD)?**—This section defines ASD and presents prevalence information.

▶ **What Challenges Exist for Diagnosing ASD?**—This section covers risk factors for PTSD, differentiating ASD from PTSD, DSM-IV diagnostic criteria, and assessing ASD in clinical interviews using assessment and diagnostic tools.

▶ **Is There a Treatment for ASD?**—This section reviews common treatment options for patients with ASD.

IMMEDIATELY after a traumatic event, those exposed may experience severe and incapacitating psychological distress. They may avoid traumatic stimuli and have startle reactions, hypervigilance, or other symptoms associated with PTSD. However, these distressing symptoms appear to be within the normal, immediate human response to overwhelming events.

Most people exposed to traumatic events never develop PTSD, depression, alcoholism, or any other *DSM-IV–TR* psychiatric disorder. A review of 160 studies on disaster victims suggests that two-thirds will not develop a clinically significant chronic psychiatric disorder.[215–217] Most reactions were transient with symptom dissipation within a month of the disaster for 42 percent of the victims, and within a year for an additional 23 percent. Only a substantial minority, 30 percent, experienced chronic symptoms lasting more than a year.

Consider the reactions of two U.S. World Trade Center disaster survivors, Kevin W. and William G.

▶ **Kevin**, who was lucky enough to flee his office in the South Tower shortly after the North Tower was hit, was not injured physically but witnessed terrifying death and destruction all around him.

▶ **William** was led from the 64th floor of the South Tower by firefighters and experienced all that Kevin had plus breathing problems from the smoke.

From the Patient's Perspective

Kevin W. or William G.—Immediate Post-Trauma Aftermath

It's been two days now, and I'm a nervous wreck. I know I should be thankful that I got out alive, but I'm climbing the walls. I jump at the slightest noise. I'm glued to the TV, and every time the instant replay shows those planes hitting the Twin Towers, I go into a panic, start to sweat, can't calm down, can't stop thinking about all those who didn't make it, and can't sleep because of the nightmares, can't stop smelling the awful smoke, and can't stop hearing the cries for help from those trapped on the upper floors.

Both were extremely distressed during the immediate post-traumatic aftermath and might characterize their feelings as in the first "From the Patient's Perspective" box on this page.

However, what they report two weeks later (in the next "From the Patient's Perspective" box) reflects symptoms that may differentiate an acute stress reaction (ASR) from an acute stress disorder (ASD).

From the Patient's Perspective

Kevin W. and William G.—Two Weeks Later

Kevin W.: Acute Stress Reaction

It's been two weeks since the Twin Towers were attacked. In the beginning, I couldn't seem to get a grip. Sally said that for the first few days, I was screaming in my sleep and thrashing about in the bed. When awake, she said, I seemed to be off somewhere else when she tried to get my attention or comfort me. Thankfully, I've moved way beyond that point and no longer have the nightmares, anxiety, or spacey feelings. Although I'll never forget what happened, things are returning to normal, and my life continues to progress beyond September 11th.

William G.: Acute Stress Disorder

It's been two weeks, and I'm still not myself. I jump at the slightest sound, can't focus on anything at work or at home, can't sleep, and can't stop thinking about how my panic got even worse when I couldn't breathe because of the thick smoke in the stairway as I frantically tried to get out of the building. And my internal world seems completely different. It's like living in a dream world instead of real life. I'm not connected to my feelings. It almost seems like I'm outside, looking in. Watching someone who looks like me but really isn't.

Most people (like Kevin W.) exposed to a traumatic event who exhibit acute stress reaction (ASR) will recover spontaneously within a few days. Only a minority will develop ASD (like William G.), or some other psychiatric problem. However, since the vast majority of people who survive a catastrophic stressor will be very distressed during the immediate postdisaster aftermath, it is usually impossible to distinguish those who are most likely to recover on their own from those at greatest risk of developing a chronic psychiatric disorder.

This chapter considers this challenge and reviews current thinking about the best approach for ameliorating normal distress and treating clinically significant problems.

Military Considerations

The current wars in Iraq and Afghanistan have resulted in PTSD among approximately 15 percent of service men and women.[220] Indeed, given the remarkable advances in military medicine and the efficiency of the medical evacuation system, only 10 percent of those wounded in battle are dying from their injuries compared to 25 percent in previous wars.[221] Higher survivor rates are no doubt one reason why psychiatric casualties have assumed such prominence. Another reason is the growth of knowledge regarding the recognition and treatment of posttraumatic reactions and disorders that has informed current military policy and practice.[222]

Acute psychological distress or functional incapacity has been a longtime concern of military and civilian psychiatry. Whereas in the civilian sector this is called ASR, in a military context it is called combat operational stress reaction (COSR). In this chapter

Within three to five days of the September 11, 2001, World Trade Center attacks, 90 percent of Americans surveyed nationally reported at least moderate distress, while 44 percent of respondents reported one or more substantial symptoms of severe distress.[218] In contrast to the high prevalence of normal posttraumatic distress, a much smaller percentage of New Yorkers, 7.5 percent, developed PTSD within weeks of the World Trade Center attacks.[219]

we will review COSR as well as ASR, since there are specific interventions (e.g., PIES and BICEPS, see below) that the military has developed that are not only important in their own right but also have greatly influenced interventions developed for civilians, such as psychological first aid.

Furthermore, the desire to make troops more resilient, and therefore less likely to develop behavioral, emotional, or psychiatric problems after exposure to traumatic events has caused military leaders to develop programs that it is hoped will produce psychological as well as physical toughness among troops preparing for deployment. The army, marines/navy, and air force have each established resilience programs to enable troops to obtain the psychological protection they need in a war zone. This development coincides with the recent growth in our scientific understanding of resilience, which is a very complicated set of attributes that has genetic, psychobiological, cognitive, emotional, behavioral, and social dimensions.[16]

Many combat injuries are caused by powerful explosions from roadside bombs and explosive devices detonated from vehicles, or rocket-propelled grenades and other explosives directed at convoys and troops. In addition to the psychological trauma of exposure to such powerful explosions (which often cause death, injury, and major destruction), servicemen and women who survive such events may also have serious head injuries. These concussive injuries are called traumatic brain injuries (TBIs), which may be mild (which is most common), moderate, or severe (which may cause serious impairment of brain function as well as blindness and other neurological losses).

Since any concussive injury serious enough to literally rattle your brain is serious enough to cause traumatic stress, it is not uncommon for PTSD and TBI to occur in the same individual at the same time. For clinicians evaluating such servicemen and women weeks, months, or years after the explosive encounter, it is often difficult to distinguish which symptoms are due to PTSD and which to TBI since there is much overlap, especially with mild TBI.[223] Since this chapter focuses on short-term evaluation and treatment, such long-term issues will not be addressed. What does seem pertinent to the present discussion, however, is that at the present time, it appears that individuals with PTSD and mild (but not moderate or severe) TBI should be offered the same interventions and treatment as those with PTSD alone. This is obviously a matter of great importance and a high-priority area for current research.

What Are Normal Acute, Posttraumatic Distress Reactions?

Identification of a person with ASR or COSR is based primarily on observation of the severity of their emotional distress and functional impairment. Acute stress reactions may present in a number of ways with different individuals exhibiting different symptoms. In addition to reexperiencing, dissociative, avoidance, and hyperarousal symptoms, people with ASR/COSR may exhibit the following symptoms for days or weeks following the trauma:

- ▶ Emotional reactions—Shock, fear, grief, anger, resentment, guilt, shame, helplessness, hopelessness, and numbing

- ▶ Cognitive reactions—Confusion, disorientation, indecisiveness, difficulty concentrating, memory loss, self-blame, and unwanted memories

- ▶ Physical reactions—Tension, fatigue, edginess, insomnia, startle reactions, racing heartbeat, nausea, loss of appetite, and change in sex drive

- ▶ Interpersonal reactions—Distrust, irritability, withdrawal, and isolation; feeling rejected or abandoned; being distant, judgmental, or overcontrolling

These reactions may vary from mild to severe. In some cases, there is evidence of more clinical symptoms, such as intrusive recollections, marked avoidance, dissociation, psychic numbing, panic attacks, intense agitation, incapacitating anxiety, severe depression, and grief reactions (over the death or injury of loved ones as well as personal material losses).

At an early stage, the appropriate professional stance is that these are transient reactions from which normal recovery should be expected.[224]

Counseling the Patient with an Acute Stress Reaction

In a first session following a traumatic event, an individual may be so distressed that the clinician will be unsure as to whether he or she will develop ASD or PTSD. Barring definitive symptoms for either disorder, preliminary counseling may involve providing educational information about acute stress reactions and recommending further contact if symptoms increase. This education typically emphasizes that what the patient is experiencing:

- ▶ Affects almost everyone exposed to catastrophic stress
- ▶ Usually resolves within days or weeks

- ▶ Typically does not lead to any permanent psychological scars or psychiatric problems

Key recommendations for these patients include:

- ▶ Avoiding reexposure to traumatic reminders (e.g., not watching traumatic images on TV)
- ▶ Spending as much time as possible with friends and family
- ▶ Being patient so that normal recovery can take place

What Treatment Approaches Are Used for Traumatic Event Survivors?

There is growing consensus that the best mental health intervention during the immediate aftermath of a traumatic event is *psychological first aid*, which would include:[225]

psychological first aid—an approach designed to ameliorate immediate posttraumatic distress based on the expectation that every survivor, no matter how upset, will achieve normal recovery

- ▶ Provision of basic needs—safety, security, and survival (food and shelter)
- ▶ Orientation to disaster and recovery efforts
- ▶ Reduction of physiological arousal through self-calming and relaxation techniques, avoiding upsetting stimuli, and (occasionally) taking medication
- ▶ Mobilization of support for those most distressed through reunion with family/friends and provision of needed professional services
- ▶ Providing education about available resources and coping strategies
- ▶ Using effective risk communication techniques to provide accurate, necessary information to survivors in a calm, honest, and straightforward manner without increasing anxiety

Following exposure to a traumatic event, individuals should be encouraged to live their lives as normally as possible and avoid isolating themselves from family, friends, or community-based natural support systems (e.g., neighborhood, school, church, or workplace organizations).

Information available through print and broadcast media, Internet sites, and toll-free telephone hotlines rank among key vehicles for carrying out such a public health approach.

In the event of a natural or man-made disaster, public health approaches in the vicinity of the terrorist attack or disaster site should have both educational and outreach components.[226] Such large-scale, community/societal interventions should be designed to promote resilience and foster recovery among the majority of the population temporarily suffering from acute posttraumatic reactions. They also need to provide widely accessible information about clinically significant posttraumatic symptoms so that people can make accurate appraisals concerning the magnitude of their own distress as well as that of loved ones and friends. Such a proactive approach should also indicate what type of mental health services might be helpful and where they can be found.

PROJECT LIBERTY

New York City's post-9/11 disaster mental health program, Project Liberty, illustrates effective media–public health partnerships that benefit the general public after a major catastrophe. A broad-scale, public media campaign such as this should have four objectives:[227]

1. Branding a disaster-response program to provide recognition of available services

2. Broadcasting the overall message that posttraumatic distress is a normal reaction

3. Promoting a sense of security for the community at large by announcing that mental health services are available to those in need

4. Identifying and legitimizing outreach staff conducting face-to-face and door-to-door outreach services

Two weeks following the attack, Project Liberty developed and aired a 30-second TV commercial directing people to available mental health services. Within two months, 25 percent of New Yorkers knew about Project Liberty, and 70 percent reported that they had learned about it through television.[227]

Project Liberty also used radio announcements, printed brochures, a toll-free phone number, and information on the Internet. In addition, the project's community-directed interventions were tailored specifically for schoolchildren, the elderly, the workplace, and for many distinct ethnic communities.[227]

Forward Psychiatry for Combat Operational Stress Reaction (COSR)

In the military, clinicians found that active duty personnel who had an incapacitating anxiety attack (e.g., "battle fatigue" or "combat operational stress reaction") had better outcomes if treated at a medical unit close to the war zone, such as a battalion aid station.[228] Thought to produce rapid resolution of battle fatigue and prevent the later development of what is now called PTSD, military psychological acute intervention (PIES) included these main components:

1. Proximity—Providing intervention at a location as close to the active combat zone as possible

2. Immediacy—Intervening as soon as possible after the onset of battle fatigue

3. Expectancy—Providing education that the acute stress reaction is a normal human response to an overwhelming and abnormal event, including the expectation that the individual will quickly recover and return to military

duties within a few days without immediate or long-term consequences from the acute stress reaction

4. Simplicity—Using brief, straightforward methods to restore physical and psychological well-being and self-confidence

Although the military PIES approach has not been rigorously tested, its apparent success fostered the use of similar interventions for civilians who experienced natural disasters or man-made catastrophes as exemplified by psychological first aid.[229]

A later version of PIES called BICEPS is currently utilized by the military.

1. Brevity—Initial rest and replenishment ("3 hots and a cot") at Combat Operation Stress Control facilities located close to the service member's unit lasting no more than 1–3 days.

2. Immediacy—Treatment begins as soon as tactically and logistically possible.

3. Contact—Service personnel are encouraged to continue to think of themselves as war fighters and not as patients or sick persons.

4. Expectancy—Explicit message that this is a normal reaction to war zone stress from which complete recovery is expected with a return to full duty in a few hours or days.

5. Proximity—If care cannot be adequately provided in the unit, it is provided at the battalion aid station or medical company nearest the unit; the locus of care is separated from that provided to medical or surgical patients.

6. Simplicity—Using brief and straightforward methods.

Approaches such as this are currently provided to U.S. military personnel in Iraq and Afghanistan to soldiers by Army Combat Stress Control (CSR) mental health units. The marines' approach is somewhat different and is provided by Operational Stress Control and Readiness (OSCAR) units. Both CSR and OSCAR approaches are evidence-informed but have yet to be tested rigorously.[224,225,229,230]

Resilience

Concern about mental fitness among fighting troops has naturally led to development of programs to foster mental toughening or resilience among troops before deployment to a war zone. It is obvious that greater resilience should result in fewer incidents of COSR and therefore significantly reduce COSR and more chronic trauma-related mental health problems among servicemen and women. As a result, the army, navy/marines, and air force have each developed resilience programs to improve psychological preparation for troops, which are currently operational.[231] The basic principles of such programs are:

1. **Provide realistic training** (with simulations, if possible) of war zone scenarios.

2. **Strengthen perceived ability to cope** with trauma and its aftermath.

3. **Create supportive interpersonal work environments** (such as increased unit cohesion) to optimize social support.

4. **Develop and maintain adaptive beliefs** about realistic expectations, confidence in leadership, confidence in the meaningfulness of the military mission, and confidence in one's own coping abilities.

5. **Develop comprehensive stress management programs** and increase awareness of their availability while reducing the stigma attached to seeking help for stress-related problems.

Understanding resilience has become one of the major challenges in the trauma field. It is a very complex construct consisting of genetic, psychobiological, cognitive, emotional, behavioral, and social aspects. Since everyone will encounter stress throughout life and more than half of us will be exposed to traumatic stress, it behooves us to learn as much about resilience as possible so that we can equip our children and ourselves (as well as our military, police, firefighter, and first responder personnel) to prepare for stress as well as possible and to have the necessary coping abilities to confront stressful/traumatic situations when they arise.[16]

Psychological Debriefing

Psychological debriefing was first developed for police, firefighters, and first responders to help them cope with the traumatic situations that they encountered on a daily basis as part of their professional responsibilities. It was later adapted by the military and utilized in the war zone. It was predicated on the assumption that the best approach for those who experience a catastrophic event is early detection and timely intervention.

Proponents of psychological debriefing assert that it can abort the onset of a serious mental disorder, can reduce severity and duration once it has taken hold, or can prevent ASR or COSR from progressing to a chronic and incapacitating PTSD or some other debilitating psychiatric disorder.

psychological debriefing— an intervention conducted by trained professionals shortly after a catastrophe, allowing victims to talk about their experience and receive information on "normal" types of reactions to such an event

The best known form of psychological debriefing is Critical Incident Stress Debriefing (CISD).[232] However, its many modifications and variations have led to use of the more general term, psychological debriefing.

Psychological debriefing is often conducted in two-hour sessions with 10–20 participants, typically following this process:[230, 232,233]

- ► The group shares facts about the traumatic event.
- ► The group collectively reviews personal thoughts, impressions, and emotional reactions.
- ► The facilitator informs participants that it is quite natural for some people to have disturbing symptoms shortly after a traumatic event.

Subsequently, group members are encouraged to speak about any such symptoms they may have experienced. Then the group focuses on effective internal coping mechanisms and external (social) support.

> *According to proponents of psychological debriefing, this sharing of such intense personal information gives participants a chance to vent powerful feelings and learn that others have had similar reactions.*
>
> *In spite of research to the contrary, most disaster survivors and clinicians who treat them feel that they benefited from the intervention. This is because most disaster survivors do not develop PTSD, whether or not they receive psychological debriefing.*

- ► The facilitator distributes psychoeducational materials describing the normal human response to catastrophic stress and debriefs the group, generating a positive expectancy that disturbing, posttraumatic stress symptoms will probably subside within weeks.
- ► Group members receive lists of available mental health practitioners to contact if their symptoms do not subside.

Psychological Debriefing Effectiveness in Preventing Later PTSD

Despite its popularity and history, research suggests that psychological debriefing recipients either receive no benefit or actually experience a worsening of their symptoms.[230,234]

Many rigorous, randomized clinical trials (RCTs) on psychological debriefing have been conducted.[230,234] In most cases, the intervention tested consisted of a single session of individual debriefing, administered within the first month after the traumatic event. In recent years, there have also been randomized trials of group debriefings among military personnel. In no case did debriefing prevent the later development of PTSD. In some cases, it appeared to delay recovery since comparison subjects who did not receive debriefing were less symptomatic at follow-up.[235,236]

Four theoretical reasons for the consistent failure (and possibly counterproductive) effect of debriefing on recovery are the following:

1. Forcing premature exposure to traumatic memories may actually interfere with a natural recovery process that allows the traumatic material to be consolidated and then to fade from conscious awareness.[230,237]

2. Debriefing during the immediate posttraumatic aftermath may actively interfere with habituation and cognitive changes that are essential for normal recovery.[337,238]

3. An early focus on acute posttraumatic symptoms may foster negative cognitions about oneself (e.g., "Most people feel better by now so there must be something wrong with me"). Negative cognitions predict the later development of PTSD.[239,240]

4. Excessive posttraumatic adrenergic activity predicts PTSD because it facilitates the encoding of traumatic memories.[241,242] Debriefing may activate such mechanisms, thereby facilitating the encoding of intrusive memories that increase the risk for PTSD.[243]

> *Avoidance may be an important adaptive strategy in the very early stages of normal recovery from traumatic events and should not be disrupted by early interventions such as debriefing.[244]*

What Is Acute Stress Disorder (ASD)?

Most people exposed to a traumatic event will exhibit psychological distress; for some, this distress will be a transient acute stress reaction that may be briefly incapacitating, at most. For others, this distress may signal the start of a severe, chronic, and potentially incapacitating psychiatric disorder. The public health problem lies in distinguishing vulnerable from resilient individuals during the immediate aftermath of a terrorist attack, mass casualty, or natural disaster. Long ago, military psychiatrists named these acute reactions "combat stress reaction" or "battle fatigue." Now it is called COSR.

> *In Stephen Crane's novel about the Civil War, The Red Badge of Courage, the protagonist, a new recruit to the Union Army, has a classic attack of an acute stress reaction during his first exposure to enemy gunfire, from which he shortly recovers.*

Although most recover from COSR, a significant minority of people will experience persistent reactions and go on to develop PTSD after a month passes. Until the *DSM-IV*, there was no recognized diagnosis that could be given to an individual suffering high-magnitude and clinically significant distress during the immediate aftermath of a traumatic event. Today, the *DSM-IV–TR* provides specific criteria for diagnosing ASD (see Figure 6.2 on page 97).

Studies conducted shortly after disasters and other traumatic events found ASD in 7 to 33 percent of survivors. More importantly, the incidence of ASD rather successfully predicts the later development of PTSD—overall, 70 to 80 percent of people with ASD will develop PTSD. However, approximately 60 percent of those who develop PTSD do so without ever meeting diagnostic criteria for ASD.[245–248]

> *Among children, only 12 percent with ASD developed PTSD at follow-up.[249]*

Early detection is important for treatment as different interventions may be indicated for people depending on their level of vulnerability vs. resilience.

What Challenges Exist for Diagnosing ASD?

Currently, the lack of empirical research into prognosis and risk factors makes differentiation extremely difficult.

Risk Factors for ASD

Although little research data on risk factors exists for ASD, they are probably similar to those related to PTSD (see Chapter 2, page 19). Peritraumatic dissociation was also considered to be a risk factor for ASD. Subsequent research, however, suggests that it is the posttraumatic persistence of dissociation, rather than the peritraumatic occurrence of dissociation that predicts ASD.[250] There are apparently many risk factors for ASD. These include ongoing life stress, lack of social support, preexisting psychiatric disorders or substance abuse, female gender (among civilian, but not military women), low education, low intelligence, childhood abuse or other adverse experiences, family history of psychiatric disorders, poor training or preparation, stress severity, depression, and an avoidant coping style.[250]

In addition, ASD has only limited usefulness as a screening criterion for the general population since most people who develop PTSD fail to meet ASD criteria beforehand.[250] This is a concern for public mental health planners who, understandably, want to neither label normal and transient posttraumatic symptoms as pathologic nor use scarce and expensive clinical resources for individuals who will recover spontaneously or with minimal assistance.

PTSD and ASD symptoms are similar in terms of reexperiencing and hyperarousal symptoms (which are identical), and ASD avoidant symptoms (which are the same as the first two avoidant/numbing symptoms for PTSD). Differences involve emphasis, number of symptoms in each category, and definition of functional impairment. Figure 6.1 provides an at-a-glance reference for these differences.

Distinguishing ASD from PTSD

The major difference between ASD and PTSD is the greater emphasis placed on symptoms of dissociation, which is characterized by normal mental functions (e.g., memory, a sense of time, or a sense of one's body or personal identity as a coherent entity) being severely distorted. To meet ASD diagnostic criteria, an acutely traumatized individual must exhibit three *dissociative* symptoms (criterion B symptoms), while it is possible to diagnose PTSD with none. These dissociative symptoms include:

1. Reduction in Awareness (Criterion B2)—An individual's perceptions, thoughts, and feelings are focused inter-

Although not sufficiently tested, prognostic indicators for the development of chronic symptoms appear to be functional impairment, elevated heart rate, and negative cognitions.[217,237,241,250]

It is the inclusion and prominence of dissociative symptoms that sets ASD distinctly apart from PTSD.

dissociation—an abnormal cognitive/emotional state in which one's perception of oneself, one's environment, or the relationship between oneself and one's environment is altered significantly.

Figure 6.1   Diagnostic Differences between ASD and PTSD

Differences	ASD	PTSD
Emphasis	Dissociative Symptoms	Avoidant and Numbing Symptoms
Number of Dissociative Symptoms	3 (including 1 numbing and 1 amnesia symptom)	0
Number of Avoidant Symptoms	1	3 (avoidant and numbing)
Number of Anxiety/Arousal Symptoms	1	2
Onset/Duration of Symptoms	2 days to 4 weeks	More than 4 weeks
Functional Impairment	Clinically significant distress and functional impairment; unable to obtain necessary assistance	Clinically significant distress and impairment socially, occupationally, and in other important areas of functioning

nally rather than on external surroundings, appearing to onlookers as the individual being "in a daze," "spaced-out," or in a world of his or her own.

2. *Derealization* (Criterion B3)—Typical perceptions of the external environment are significantly altered. One's sense of time may be accelerated or slowed down. People or objects appear to have lost their substance. The world one has always known is dramatically changed, and one feels estranged or detached from the environment or has a sense that the environment is unreal. For example, one may feel that familiar, routine places seem unfamiliar.

3. *Depersonalization* (Criterion B4)—It appears that one's self, rather than one's world (as in derealization), has changed. Depersonalization may manifest itself as a distorted perception of one's body, identity, or self as a coherent entity (e.g., having an out-of-body experience of looking down on one's body from above; or feeling that one's body is split into sections: one part might be numb, another warm, and another cold).

4. Numbing (Criterion B1)—In ASD, PTSD numbing symptoms (C5–6), detachment and psychic numbing, are considered one (of five) dissociative symptom clusters.

5. Amnesia (Criterion B5)—Likewise, in ASD, PTSD amnesia (C3) is considered a dissociative symptom.

In addition to dissociative symptoms, ASD must last a minimum of two days and a maximum of four weeks, whereas PTSD

derealization—an alteration in the perception or experience of the external world so that it seems strange or unreal (e.g., people may seem unfamiliar or mechanical)

depersonalization—an alteration in the perception or experience of the self so that one feels detached from, and as if one is an outside observer of, one's mental processes or body (e.g., feeling as if one is in a dream) cannot be diagnosed until at least four weeks after the traumatic experience.

Understanding *DSM-IV* Diagnostic Criteria

ASD is a diagnostic classification for people experiencing significant psychological distress within one month of a trauma. Figure 6.2, on page 97, presents the *DSM-IV–TR* diagnostic criteria for ASD.

See page 12 for complete diagnostic criteria of PTSD.

Conducting a Clinical Interview for ASD

The caution, sensitivity, and patience a clinician uses in a PTSD diagnostic interview must also be evident to the patient during an ASD assessment. The major difference, of course, is that the PTSD patient has a chronic condition to which the patient has had an opportunity to adapt, whereas ASD patients have been acutely traumatized, finding themselves in an intense, novel, and extremely disturbing psychological state difficult to comprehend. Patients may feel they are out of control and/or as if they are losing their minds, perhaps exhibiting severe anxiety, agitation, and apprehension. Therefore, when conducting an ASD assessment, the clinician must initially approach it as carefully and thoughtfully as any other urgent or emergent psychiatric evaluation.

ASD Assessment and Diagnostic Tools

ASD instruments can be used to assess both diagnosis and symptom severity. PTSD trauma exposure scales will also serve to determine Criterion A for ASD. There are three standardized assessment instruments for ASD.

The Acute Stress Disorder Interview (ASDI)[250] consists of 19 "yes/no" questions, each representing one of the ASD diagnostic criteria. Symptom severity is assessed by adding up the number of "yes" responses.

The Acute Stress Disorder Scale (ASDS)[252] consists of a 5-point Likert scale for each of the 19 ASD items. It therefore provides a more fine-grained assessment of ASD symptom severity, much like the PCL and PSS for PTSD.

The Stanford Acute Stress Reaction Questionnaire (SASRQ)[253] is a 30-item self-report Likert scale that enquires about dissociative, somatic, reexperiencing, hyperarousal, insomnia, and cognitive symptoms.

Figure 6.2 *DSM-IV-TR* Diagnostic Criteria for Acute Stress Disorder[5]

A. The person has been exposed to a traumatic event in which both of the following were present:

   1. the person experienced, witnessed, or was confronted with an event or events that involved actual or threatened death or serious injury, or a threat to the physical integrity of self or others

   2. the person's response involved intense fear, helplessness, or horror

B. Either while experiencing or after experiencing the distressing event, the individual has three (or more) of the following dissociative symptoms:

   1. a subjective sense of numbing, detachment, or absence of emotional responsiveness

   2. a reduction in awareness of his or her surroundings (e.g., "being in a daze")

   3. derealization

   4. depersonalization

   5. dissociative amnesia (i.e., inability to recall an important aspect of the trauma)

C. The traumatic event is persistently reexperienced in at least one of the following ways: recurrent images, thoughts, dreams, illusions, flashback episodes, or a sense of reliving the experience; or distress on exposure to reminders of the traumatic event.

D. Marked avoidance of stimuli that arouse recollections of the trauma (e.g., thoughts, feelings, conversations, activities, places, people).

E. Marked symptoms of anxiety or increased arousal (e.g., difficulty sleeping, irritability, poor concentration, hypervigilance, exaggerated startle response, motor restlessness).

F. The disturbance causes clinically significant distress or impairment in social, occupational, or other important areas of functioning or impairs the individual's ability to pursue some necessary task, such as obtaining necessary assistance or mobilizing personal resources by telling family members about the traumatic experience.

G. The disturbance lasts for a minimum of 2 days and a maximum of 4 weeks and occurs within 4 weeks of the traumatic event.

H. The disturbance is not due to the direct physiological effects of a substance (e.g., a drug of abuse, a medication) or a general medical condition, is not better accounted for by Brief Psychotic Disorder, and is not merely an exacerbation of a preexisting Axis I or Axis II disorder.

Empirical justification for including these three dissociative symptoms for ASD is sparse. It relies mostly on clinical observations and on evidence showing that people who experience acute dissociative symptoms during a traumatic event are at a greater risk for later developing PTSD.

Source: Reprinted with permission by the American Psychiatric Association: *Diagnostic and Statistical Manual of Mental Disorders, Fourth Edition Text Revision.* Washington, DC: American Psychiatric Association, 2000.

Is There a Treatment for ASD?

Cognitive-Behavioral Therapy

In contrast to negative findings with debriefing, a number of RCTs testing CBT have had very promising results. These brief CBT interventions are usually not initiated until at least 14 days after traumatic exposure, much later than the standard 4-day, posttraumatic window in which psychological first aid should be offered.

See pages 43–51 for a detailed description of CBT.

Brief CBT protocols of four or five sessions that include both exposure therapy and cognitive restructuring have been shown to ameliorate ASD and to effectively reduce the subsequent development of PTSD. Brief CBT also appears to be more effective than supportive counseling, self-help, repeated assessment, or a naturalistic control group.[254–257]

Pharmacological Treatments and Acute Distress

Given abundant evidence that excessive noradrenergic activity is associated with PTSD, and because it may increase the likelihood of developing intrusive, emotionally arousing memories, one might expect that acute suppression of adrenergic activity would ameliorate acute posttraumatic distress and prevent PTSD.[175,243] In the only RCT testing this hypothesis, Pitman et al. reported promising but somewhat inconclusive results with the adrenergic beta-blocking agent propranolol administered to accident victims within six hours of the event.[258] Two other reports also suggest that propranolol may be an effective treatment for acutely traumatized individuals.[259,260] Based on the inconclusiveness of current evidence, propranolol cannot be recommended as a prophylactic agent to prevent the later development of PTSD. Perhaps future research will demonstrate its efficacy.

Other studies utilizing hydrocortisone acutely in intensive care or cardiac care hospital wards also had favorable results.[178] This approach has yet to be tested in emergency room or other settings before it can be recommended for general use.

The most exciting finding is a recent report regarding acute morphine administration to navy and marine personnel wounded in Iraq and evacuated (usually within 1–3 hours) to a battalion aid station. Wounded servicemen who received acute morphine administration had significantly lower rates of PTSD when assessed several months later than those who did not receive morphine. Whether this finding can be replicated and whether the success of morphine was due to rapid pain reduction, antagonism of noradrenergic activity, or both, remains to be seen.[261]

Treating Acutely Traumatized Children

At present, no empirical evidence exists to support any early intervention for children. As with adults who may have had an adverse reaction to psychological debriefing, there are salient reasons to be concerned about premature interventions with children and adolescents.[262,263] Information on the effectiveness of treatment for children is largely based on CBT trials for chronic PTSD.

Since young children base their perceptions of events on their parents' perceptions and behavior (i.e., social referencing), children may perceive that they are still in danger and become more symptomatic if their parents continue to exhibit high levels of posttraumatic distress.

One RCT on early intervention with pharmacotherapy involved recently traumatized children on a burn unit with ASD in which the tricyclic antidepressant imipramine produced greater reduction in ASD symptoms than the sedative/hypnotic chloral-hydrate.[264] Unfortunately, a recent replication of this study by the same investigators found that neither imipramine nor fluoxetine was superior to placebo in reducing ASD symptoms.[265] In a naturalistic study with pediatric burn victims, acute morphine administration during hospitalization prevented the later development of PTSD symptoms.[266]

> *To date, there are no empirical studies of psychosocial interventions for children and adolescents implemented within the first month after a traumatic event, nor is there information about the effectiveness of pharmacology or what dosage may be most effective.*
>
> *Opiates inhibit neuronal activity in the amygdala and antagonize the actions of CRF and adrenergic neurotransmitters.*

Key Concepts for Chapter 6

1. Research indicates that as many as two-thirds of disaster victims never develop PTSD or other psychiatric disorders as a result. Many, however, will experience transient reactions that typically dissipate within a month of the traumatic event and are categorized as acute stress reactions.

2. Acute stress disorder (ASD) is a condition characterized by more dissociative symptoms than avoidant or arousal ones. These symptoms include being focused internally and less aware of external surroundings, having significantly altered perceptions of the external environment (derealization), and having a distorted perception of one's body or identity.

3. Key recommendations for those experiencing acute stress reactions include avoiding reexposure to traumatic reminders, spending extensive time with supportive friends and family, and patiently allowing normal recovery to occur.

4. Interventions immediately after a traumatic event should include providing for basic needs, orienting oneself to the disaster and the recovery efforts, reducing psychophysiological arousal, mobilizing support for those most distressed, getting and keeping families together, educating victims about support strategies and resources, and effectively communicating risk without engendering more anxiety.

5. Military psychiatry and psychology has been in the forefront of developing acute interventions for acutely traumatized servicemen and women with Combat Operational Stress Reactions. These include development of the PIES (proximity, immediacy, expectancy, and simplicity) and BICEPS (brevity, immediacy, contact, expectancy, proximity, and simplicity) approaches.

6. An emphasis on resilience has become a major priority in both military and civilian public health sectors.

7. There is no evidence that psychological debriefing is effective. Psychological first aid appears to be a more effective approach during the immediate aftermath of a large-scale traumatic event, but it has not been tested rigorously.

8. As with PTSD, CBT has proven most effective for those with ASD. Research on pharmacological interventions has not identified effective medications that prevent the later development of PTSD or that ameliorate the symptoms of ASD.

9. No empirical evidence exists indicating that early intervention is effective with acutely traumatized children; however, psychological first aid is developmentally sensitive and has been designed for this purpose. There may be a major benefit to ensuring that parents do not experience high levels of posttraumatic distress that could lead children to believe that there is a risk of additional trauma.

Appendix

Appendix Table 1   Screening Instruments

SCALE	FULL NAME	#ITEMS	USE	REFERENCE
PC-PTSD	Primary Care PTSD Screen	4	Primary Care VA and DoD Surveys	267
TSQ	Trauma Screening Questionnaire	10	Disasters and Emergency Rooms	268
SIPS	Single Item PTSD Screen	1	Primary Care	269

VA = Department of Veterans Affairs
DoD = Department of Defense

Appendix Table 2   Trauma Exposure Scales for Adults

	Instrument	Self-Report	Structured Interview	Reference
General	Traumatic Stress Schedule (TSS)	X		270
	Potential Stressor Experiences Inventory (PSEI)	X		271
	Traumatic Events Questionnaire (TEQ)	X		272
	Evaluation of Lifetime Stressors (ELS)		X	273
	The Trauma History Questionnaire (THQ)	X		274
	Traumatic Life Events Questionnaire (TLEQ)	X		275
	Stressful Life Events Screening Questionnaire (SLESQ)	X		276
	Life Stressor Checklist—Revised (LSC-R)	X		277
Childhood Trauma	Child Abuse and Trauma Scale	X		278
	Childhood Trauma Questionnaire	X		279
	Familial Experiences Inventory		X	280
	Retrospective Assessment of Traumatic Experiences (RATE)	X		281
	Early Trauma Inventory (ETI)		X	282
Domestic Violence	Conflict Tactics Scale (CTS)	X		283
	Abusive Behavior Inventory (ABI)	X		284
	Sexual Experiences Survey (SES)	X		285
	Wyatt Sex History Questionnaire (WSHQ)		X	286
Zone Trauma	Combat Exposure Scale (CES)	X		287
	Women's Wartime Stressor Scale (WWSS)	X		288
Torture	Harvard Trauma Questionnaire (HTQ)	X		289

Appendix Table 3 PTSD Diagnostic Instruments for Adults

Scale	Full Name	Diagnostic	Sx Severity	Administration	Main Use	Comments	Reference
SCID.IV	Structured Interview for DSM-IV	X		CI (Clinician Interviewer)	Clinical	All DSM-IV Diagnoses assessed	290
CAPS	Clinician Administered PTSD Scale	X	X	CI	Clinical	PTSD Sx: Intensity and frequency	291
PSS-I	PTSD Symptom Scale Interview	X	X	CI	Clinical	Combined Sx severity/frequency	292
SI-PTSD	Structured Interview for PTSD	X	X	CI	Clinical	Symptom severity	293
ADIS-R	Anxiety Disorders Interview Schedule—Revised	X	X	CI	Clinical	All DSM-IV Diagnoses	294
PTSD-I	PTSD-Interview	X	X	LI (Lay Interviewer)	Clinical	Symptom severity	295
CIDI	Composite International Diagnostic Interview	X		LI	Survey	All DSM-IV Diagnoses	296
DIS-IV	Diagnostic Interview Schedule-IV	X		LI	Survey	All DSM-IV Diagnoses	297
PCL	PTSD Checklist	X	X	Self	Clinical/survey	Symptom Severity	298
PDS	Posttraumatic Stress Diagnostic Scale	X	X	Self	Clinical	Symptom Severity	299
DTS	Davidson Trauma Scale	X	X	Self	Clinical	Symptom Severity	300
DAPS	Detailed Assessment of Traumatic Stress	X	X	Self	Clinical	Sx Severity	301

Appendix Table 4   PTSD Self-Report Instruments for Adults

Scale	Full Name	Sx Severity	Diagnostic	# Items	Comments	Reference
PCL	PTSD Check List	X	X	17	Used very widely for clinical and survey research	298
PDS	Posttraumatic Stress Diagnostic Scale	X	X	17	Used extensively in treatment research	299
DTS	Davidson Trauma Scale	X	X	17	Used in medication trials	300
DAPS	Detailed Assessment of Traumatic Stress	X	X	104	Comprehensive measure of trauma and PTSD	301
IES-R	Impact of Event Scale-Revised	X		22	Does not directly correspond to diagnostic criteria	302
M-PTSD	Mississippi Scale for Combat-Related PTSD	X		35	Does not directly correspond to DSM-IV criteria; civilian version has not performed as well	303
PK-MMPI-2	Keane PTSD Scale of MMPI-2	X		47	Subscale of MMPI-2	304
TSC	Trauma Symptom Checklist	X		40	Used with adult survivors of childhood sexual abuse	305
TSI	Trauma Symptom Inventory	X		100	Expands TSC with 10 subscales to anxiety, depression, anger, PTSD, dissociation, and sexual concerns/behavior	306
Penn	Penn Inventory	X		26	Used with both veterans and civilians	307
DEQ	Distressing Event Questionnaire	X		34	Also assesses guilt, anger, and grief	308

Appendix Table 5   Trauma Exposure Scales for Children and Adolescents

Tool	Self-Report	Structured Clinical Interview	Reference
My Worst Experience Survey (MWES) and My Worst School Experience Survey (MWSES)		X	309
Traumatic Event Screening Instrument for Children (TESI-C)		X	310
When Bad Things Happen Scale (WBTHS)	X		311
Children's Sexual Behavior Inventory 3 (CSBI-3)		X*	312
Child Rating Scales of Exposure to Interpersonal Abuse (CRS-EIA)		X	313
The Angie/Andy CRS (A/A CRS)		X	314

*Administered by parents or primary caregivers

Appendix Table 6   PTSD Diagnostic Instruments for Children and Adolescents

Scale	Full Name	Diagnostic	Sx Severity	Administration	Comment	Reference
DICA-12	Diagnostic Interview for Children and Adolescents Revised	X		LI (Lay Interviewer)	Used for clinical and survey research	315
CAPS-CA	Clinician Administered PTSD Scale for Children and Adolescents	X	X	CI (Clinician Interviewer)	PTSD Sx: intensity and frequency	316
DISC	Diagnostic Interview Schedule for Children	X		LI	Survey research	317
CPTSDI	Children's PTSD Inventory	X	X	CI	Trauma exposure, PTSD Sx, and functional impairment	318
UCLA-PTSD R1	UCLA PTSD Reaction Index	X	X	Self	Assesses PTSD and Sx severity	319
K-SADS-PL	Kiddie Schedule for Affective Disorders and Schizophrenia—Present and Lifetime Version	X		CI	Assess present and lifetime PTSD	320
PTSD-SI	PTSD Semistructured Interview	X		CI	Child and parent interviewed	321

Appendix Table 7   PTSD Self-Report Instruments for Children and Adolescents

Scale	Full Name	Ages	# Items	Comments	Reference
UCLA-PTSD-RI	UCLA-PTSD Reaction Index	6–17	22	Assesses PTSD diagnosis and symptom severity	319
IES-R	Impact of Event Scale—Revised	≥7	22	Does not directly correspond to PTSD criteria	302
PTSS-C	Posttraumatic Stress Symptoms in Children	6–18	30	Used in chaotic disaster contexts	322
TSCC	Trauma Symptom Checklist for Children	8–16	54	Assesses PTSD, anxiety, depression, and anger	323
TSCYC	Trauma Symptom Checklist for Young Children	3–12	90	Completed by caregiver	324
CPSS	Child PTSD Symptom Scale	8–18	24	Assess PTSD symptoms and functional impairment	325
CROPS/PROPS	Child Report of Posttraumatic Symptoms/Parent Report of Posttraumatic Symptoms	5–14	25/30	Broad ranges of posttraumatic symptoms both from child's and parents' perspectives	326
PTSDPAC	PTSD Symptoms in Preschool-Age Children	3–5	18	Completed by caregiver	327
CBCL	Child Behavior Checklist—PTSD Subscale	4–18	13	Completed by caregiver	328

Glossary

A

adrenergic response—neuronal activation mediated by either norepinephrine (noradrenaline) or epinephrine (adrenaline)

affect lability—rapid and unpredictable shifts in mood state

amnesia—mental syndrome characterized by partial or complete memory loss

amygdala—principal nucleus in the brain for appraising emotional input and threatening stimuli

anxiolytics—medications that relieve anxiety

ataques de nervios—a common symptom of distress among Hispanic American groups involving anxiety, uncontrollable shouting and crying, trembling, heart palpitations, difficulty breathing, dizziness, fainting spells, and dissociative symptoms (e.g., amnesia and alteration of consciousness)

B

benzodiazepine family of drugs—a very effective and widely prescribed class of medications for anxiety that includes diazepam, lorazepam, alprazolam, and clonazepam

borderline personality disorder—a personality disorder characterized by extreme instabilities fluctuating between normal functioning and psychic disability

C

calor—a stress-related syndrome observed among Salvadoran women described as a surge of intense heat that may rapidly spread throughout the entire body for a few moments or for several days

cognitive-behavioral approaches—therapeutic approaches derived from conditioning and cognitive models to extinguish fear conditioning and correct erroneous cognitions, respectively

comorbid disorders—major psychiatric disorders that are present at the same time an individual has full-fledged PTSD

cortisol—a hormone produced by the adrenal cortex that plays a prominent role in the human stress response; it increases energy by raising blood glucose levels, decreases immune processes, and causes other metabolic and neurobiological actions

countertransference—a psychoanalytic term referring to the clinician's personal psychological reaction to something the patient said or did

D

depersonalization—an alteration in the perception or experience of the self so that one feels detached from one's mental processes or body as if one is an outside observer

derealization—an alteration in the perception or experience of the external world so that it seems strange or unreal (e.g., people may seem unfamiliar or mechanical)

dissociation—an abnormal cognitive/emotional state in which one's perception of oneself, one's environment, or the relationship between oneself and one's environment is altered significantly

dissociative identity disorder—previously called multiple personality disorder, which is characterized by one's personality becoming so fragmented that pronounced changes in behavior and reactivity are noticed between different social situations or social roles

E

extrapyramidal—part of the brain's cortical neuronal system that activates muscle tone and motor movement; unwanted extrpyramidal effects (such as uncontrollable involuntary motor movements or excessive rigidity) are sometimes produced by antipsychotic medications

F

fragmented thoughts—the inability to sustain continuity and coherence in one's cognitive processes

G

generalized anxiety disorder—a psychiatric disorder marked by unrealistic worry, apprehension, and uncertainty as well as physical symptoms, such as: muscle tension, restlessness, dry mouth, and frequent urination

H

hallucination—a compelling perceptual experience of seeing, hearing, or smelling something that is not actually present

hematopoietic—referring to the bone marrow's capacity to produce red and white blood cells

hyperreactive psychophysiological state—a state in which emotions are heightened and aroused and even minor events may produce a state in which the heart pounds rapidly, muscles are tense, and there is great overall agitation

hypervigilance—preoccupied by watchful or protective behavior motivated by excessive fears for personal safety

hypothalamic-pituitary-adrenocortical (HPA) axis—three anatomic structures that participate collectively in the hormonal response to stress: the hypothalamus (in the brain), the pituitary gland (a gland just below the brain), and the outer layer (cortex) of the adrenal gland

I

imaginal exposure—systematically assisting trauma survivors to confront distressing trauma memories though the use of mental imagery

in-vivo exposure—patients practice techniques learned in therapy in the environment that represents their most-feared situation

L

lifetime PTSD—those who developed PTSD at any time in their lives

N

neurotransmitters—chemical messengers that transmit signals from one nerve cell to another to elicit physiological responses

neutrality—a psychoanalytic technique by which clinicians reveal as little of themselves as possible so that thoughts, memories, and feelings generated during therapy come from the patient's intrapsychic processes rather than from an interpersonal relationship between patient and clinician

P

panic disorder—a psychiatric disorder marked by intense anxiety and panic as well as many physical symptoms, such as palpitations, shortness of breath, dizziness, sweating, and a sense of impending death

pathological changes—changes resulting in an abnormal condition that prevents proper psychological functioning

peritraumatic dissociation—dissociation during and shortly after the trauma

personality pathology—maladaptive pattern of relating to other people that severely impairs social functioning and adaptive potential

pharmacological probe—a drug that can activate psychobiological mechanisms involved in the stress response

physiological reactivity—quickening of the heart rate, blood pressure, and breathing, resulting from exposure to internal or external cues that symbolize or resemble an aspect of the traumatic event

physioneurosis—an historical designation for the clinically significant physiological as well as psychological changes observed (during the 1940s by Abram Kardiner) among veterans with "war neurosis" syndrome

postsynaptic neuron—the downstream neuron that is the target of neurotransmission

presynaptic neuron—the neuron that initiates neurotransmission by releasing the neurotransmitter into the synaptic cleft

psychic balance—a psychoanalytic term referring to the dynamic equilibrium state between those thoughts, feelings, memories, and urges the conscious mind can tolerate and those it cannot

psychic numbing—the inability to feel any emotions, either positive (love and pleasure) or negative (fear or guilt), also described as an "emotional anesthesia"

psychodynamic approaches—therapeutic approaches that focus on unconscious and conscious motivations and drives

psychogenic amnesia—the inability to remember emotionally charged events for psychological rather than neurological reasons

psychological debriefing—an intervention conducted by trained professionals shortly after a catastrophe, allowing victims to talk about their experience and receive information on "normal" types of reactions to such an event

psychological first aid—an approach designed to ameliorate immediate posttraumatic distress based on the expectation that every survivor, no matter how upset, will achieve normal recovery

psychological probe—a visual or auditory stimulus reminiscent of a traumatic experience to which a person with PTSD is exposed

psychometric instruments—tests that measure psychological factors, such as personality, intelligence, beliefs, and fears

R

receptors—membrane-bound protein molecules with a highly specific shape that facilitate binding by neurotransmitters or medications

repression—a psychoanalytic hypothetical, unconscious process by which unacceptable (often trauma-related) thoughts and feelings are kept out of conscious awareness

S

saccadic eye movements— rapid intermittent eye movement, such as that which occurs when the eyes fix on one point after another in the visual field

schizophrenia—a major psychiatric disorder characterized by disorganization and fragmentation of thought, delusions, hallucinations, apathy, disturbance of language and communication, and withdrawal from social interaction

secondary traumatization—feelings, personal distress, and symptoms sometimes evoked in people who live with an individual with PTSD

self-cohesion—knowledge and integration of previously unconscious motivations

somatization—the expression of emotional distress through physical symptoms such as peptic ulcer, headache, asthma, or chronic pain

startle reactions—"jumpy" behavior manifested as a tendency to exhibit an exaggerated startle response to unexpected noises or movements by others

Subjective Units of Distress Scale—a scale ranging from 10 to 100 with 10 being the least anxiety provoking and 100 being the most anxiety provoking; the SUDS scoring system allows the patient to express (during CBT treatment) exactly how upsetting or distressing certain stimuli are in comparison to other anxiety experiences

sympathetic nervous system—part of the autonomic nervous system that regulates arousal functions such as heart rate and blood flow

synaptic cleft—the space between one neuron and the next that must be traversed by neurotransmitters

T

teratogenic—producing fetal abnormalities during pregnancy

V

vicarious traumatization—feelings, personal distress, and symptoms that are sometimes evoked in clinicians working with PTSD patients

W

well encapsulated—psychological buffers that prevent a person from experiencing current distress from a previous traumatic event

References

1. Kessler, R.C., Sonnega, A., Bromet, E., Hughes, M., & Nelson, C.B. (1995). Posttraumatic stress disorder in the National Comorbidity Survey. *Arch Gen Psychiatry, 52*, 1048–1060.

2. De Jong, J.T.V.M., Komproe, I.H., Van Ommeren, M., El Masri, M., Mesfin, A., Khaled, N., et al. (2001). Lifetime events and posttraumatic stress disorder in 4 postconflict settings. *Journal of the American Medical Association, 286*, 555–562.

3. American Psychiatric Committee on Nomenclature and Statistics, ed. (1980). *Diagnostic and statistical manual of mental disorders* (3rd ed.). Washington, DC: American Psychiatric Association.

4. American Psychiatric Association. (1994). *Diagnostic and statistical manual of mental disorders* (4th ed.). Washington, DC: American Psychiatric Association.

5. American Psychiatric Association. (2000). *Diagnostic and statistical manual of mental disorders* (4th ed., text rev.). Washington, DC: American Psychiatric Association.

6. Mueser, K. Personal communication. June 26, 2003.

7. van der Kolk, B.A., Weisaeth, L., & van der Hart, O. (1996). History of trauma in psychiatry. In B.A. van der Kolk, A.C. McFarlane, & L. Weisaeth (Eds.), *Traumatic stress: The effects of overwhelming experience on mind, body, and society* (pp. 47–74). New York/London: Guilford Press.

8. Cohen, M.E., White, P.D., & Johnson, R.E. (1948). Neurocirculatory asthenia, anxiety neurosis, or the effort syndrome. *Arch Intern Med, 81*, 260–281.

9. Trimble, M.R. (1985). Post-traumatic stress disorder: History of a concept. In C.R. Figley (Ed.), *Trauma and its wake: Volume 1: The study and treatment of post-traumatic stress disorder* (pp. 5–14). New York: Brunner/Mazel.

10. Kardiner, A. (1941). *The traumatic neurosis of war.* New York: Hoeber.

11. Schnurr, P.P. (1991). PTSD and combat-related psychiatric symptoms in older veterans. *PTSD Research Quarterly, 2*, 1–6.

12. Schnurr, P.P., & Green, B.L. (Eds.). (2004). *Trauma and health: Physical health consequences of exposure to extreme stress.* Washington, DC: American Psychological Association.

13. Friedman, M.J. (2005). Every crisis is an opportunity. *CNS Spectrums, 10*, 96–98.

14. Green, B.L., Friedman, M.J., de Jong, J., Solomon, S., Keane, T., Fairbank, J.A., et al. (2003). *Trauma interventions in war and peace: Prevention, practice, and policy.* Amsterdam: Kluwer Academic/Plenum.

15. Friedman, M.J. (2002). Future pharmacotherapy for post-traumatic stress disorder: Prevention and treatment. *Psychiatric Clinics of North America, 25*, 427–441.

16. Southwick, S.M., Litz, B.T., Charney, D.S., & Friedman, M.J. (in press). *Comprehensive textbook on resilience.* Cambridge,UK: Cambridge University Press.

17. Friedman, M.J., & Rosenheck, R.A. (1996). PTSD as a persistent mental illness. In S. Soreff (Ed.), *The seriously and persistently mentally ill: The state-of-the-art treatment handbook* (pp. 369–389). Seattle, WA: Hogrefe & Huber.

18. Brewin, C.R., Andrews, B., & Valentine, J.D. (2000). Meta-analysis of risk factors for posttraumatic stress disorder in trauma-exposed adults. *Journal of Consulting and Clinical Psychology, 68*, 748–766.

19. Vogt, D.S., King, D.W., & King, L.A. (2007). Risk pathways for PTSD: Making sense of the literature. In M.J. Friedman, T.M. Keane, & P.A. Resick (Eds.), *Handbook of PTSD: Science and practice* (pp. 99–115). New York: Guilford.

20. Caspi, A., Sugden, K., Moffitt, T.E., Taylor, A., Craig, I.W., Harrington, H., et al. (2003). Influence of life stress on depression: Moderation by a polymorphism in the 5HTT gene. *Science, 301*, 386–389.

21. True, W., & Pitman, R.K. (1999). Genetics and posttraumatic stress disorder. In P.A. Saigh & J.D. Bremner (Eds.), *Posttraumatic stress disorder: A comprehensive text* (pp. 144–159). Boston: Allyn & Bacon.

22. Wilson, J.P., & Keane, T.M. (Eds.). (2004). *Assessing psychological trauma and PTSD* (2nd ed.). New York: Guilford.

23. Stein, M.B., & McAllister, T.W. (2009). Exploring the convergency of posttraumatic stress disorder and mild traumatic brain injury. *American Journal of Psychiatry, 166,* 768–776.

24. Friedman, M.J., & McEwen, B. (2004). PTSD, health, and allostatic load. In P.P. Schnurr & B.L. Green (Eds.), *Trauma and health: Physical health consequences of exposure to extreme stress* (pp 157–188). Washington, DC: American Psychological Association.

25. Schnurr, P.P., Friedman, M.J., & Rosenberg, S.D. (1993). Premilitary MMPI scores as predictors of combat-related PTSD symptoms. *Am J Psychiatry, 150*, 479–483.

26. Stein, M.B., Walker, J.R., Hazen, A.L., & Forde, D.R. (1997). Full and partial posttraumatic stress disorder: Findings from a community survey. *Am J Psychiatry, 154*, 1114–1119.

27. Weiss, D.S., Marmar, C.R., Schlenger, W.E., Fairbank, J.A., Jordan, B.K., Hough, R.L., et al., (1992). The prevalence of lifetime and partial post-traumatic stress disorder in Vietnam theater veterans. *J Trauma Stress, 5*, 365–376.

28. Herman, J.L. (1992). Complex PTSD: A syndrome in survivors of prolonged and repeated trauma. *J Traumatic Stress, 5*, 377–391.

29. Linehan, M.M., Tutek, D.A., Heard, H.L., & Armstrong, H.E. (1994). Interpersonal outcome of cognitive behavioral treatment for chronically suicidal borderline patients. *American Journal of Psychiatry, 151*, 1771–1776.

30. Foa, E.B., & Rothbaum, B.O. (1997). *Treating the trauma of rape: A cognitive-behavioral therapy for PTSD*. New York: Guilford.

31. Lindy, J.D. (1993). Focal psychoanalytic psychotherapy. In J.P. Wilson & B. Raphael (Eds.), *The international handbook of traumatic stress syndromes*. New York: Plenum Press.

32. Horowitz, M.J. (1986). *Stress response syndromes* (2nd ed.). New York: Jason Aronson.

33. Foa, E.B., Keane, T.M., Friedman, M.J., & Cohen, J.A. (Eds) (2009). *Effective treatments for PTSD:Practice guidelines from the International Society for Traumatic Stress Studies* (2nd ed.). New York: Guilford.

34. Ursano, R.J., Bell, C.C., Eth, S, Friedman, M.J., Norwood, A.E., Pfefferbaum, B., et al.; American Psychiatric Association Work Group on ASD and PTSD; American Psychiatric Association Steering Committee on Practice Guidelines. (2004). *Practice guidelines for the treatment of acute stress and post-traumatic stress disorder.* Washington: American Psychiatric Association.

35. *The VA/DoD Clinical Practice Guideline Working Group (2010). Management of Posttraumatic Stress Disorder.* (2010). Washington, DC, Office of Quality and Performance, U.S. Departments of Veterans Affairs and Defense. Retrieved from http://www.oqp.med.va.gov/cpg/PTS/PTS_base.htm.

36. Cohen, J.A., Bukstein, O., Walter, H., Benson, R.S., Christman, A., Farchione, T.I., et al. (2010). Practice parameter for the assessment and treatment of posttraumatic stress disorder in children and adolescents. *Journal of the American Academy of Child and Adolescents*, 49, 414–430.

37. Australian Centre for Mental Health (2007). *Australian guidelines for the treatment of adults with acute stress disorder and posttraumatic stress disorder.* Melbourne, Victoria: ACPMH.

38. Institute of Medicine. (2007). *Treatment of PTSD: Assessment of the Evidence.* Washington, DC: The National Academies Press.

39. Rothbaum, B.O., Cahill, S.P., Foa, E.G., Davidson, J.R.T., Comptom, J., Connor, K.M., et al. (2006). Augmentation of sertraline with prolonged exposure in the treatment of PTSD. *Journal of Traumatic Stress,* 17, 213–222.

40. Davis, M., Ressler, K., Rothbaum, B.O., & Richardson, R. (2006) Effects of D-cycloserine on extinction: Translation from the treatment of posttraumatic stress disorder. *Biological Psychiatry* 60, 369–375.

41. Friedman, M.J.,Cohen, J.A., Foa, E.B., & Keane, T.M. (2009). Integration and summary. In E.B. Foa, T.M. Keane, M.J. Friedman & J.A. Cohen (Eds.), *Effective treatments for PTSD: Practice guidelines from the International Society for Traumatic Stress Studies* (2nd ed., pp. 617–642). New York: Guilford.

42. Kofoed, L., Friedman, M.J., & Peck, R. (1993). Alcoholism and drug abuse in patients with PTSD. *Psychiatric Quarterly, 64,* 151–171.

43. Najavits, L.M. (2007). Psychosocial treatments for posttraumatic stress disorder. In P.E. Nathan & J.M. Gorman (Eds.), *A guide to treatments that work* (3rd ed., pp. 513–529). New York, Oxford University Press.

44. Koerner, K., & Linehan, M.M. (2000). Research on dialectical behavior therapy for patients with borderline personality disorder. *Psychiatr Clin North Am, 23,* 151–167.

45. Osterman, J.E., & de Jong, J.T.V.M. (2007). Cultural issues and trauma. In M.J. Friedman, T.M. Keane, & P.A. Resick (Eds.), *Handbook of PTSD: Science and practice* (pp. 425–446). New York, Guilford.

46. Kinzie, D. (1989). Therapeutic approaches to traumatized Cambodian refugees. *Journal of Traumatic Stress, 2,* 75–91.

47. Stamm, B.H., & Friedman, M.J. (1999). Transcultural perspectives on post-traumatic stress disorder and other reactions to extreme stress. In A. Shalev, R. Yehuda, & A. McFarlane (Eds.), *Human response to trauma across cultural, gender, and life course* (pp. 69–85). New York: Plenum Press.

48. Marsella, A.J., Friedman, M.J., Gerrety, E.T. & Scurfield, R.M. (1996). *Ethnocultural aspects of post-traumatic stress disorder: Issues, research and clinical applications.* Washington, DC: American Psychological Association

49. Roth, S., & Friedman, M.J. (Eds.). (1998). *Childhood trauma remembered: A report on the current scientific knowledge base and its applications.* Northbrook, IL: International Society for Traumatic Stress Studies.

50. Williams, L.M. (1994). Recall of childhood trauma: A prospective study of women's memories of child sexual abuse. *Journal of Consulting and Clinical Psychology, 62*, 1167–1176.

51. Herman, J.L., & Schatzow, E. (1987). Recovery and verification of memories of childhood sexual trauma. *Psychoanal Psychol, 4*, 1–14.

52. Schacter, D.L. (1996). *Search for memory*. New York: Basic Books.

53. Lindsay, D.S., & Read, J.D. (1994). Psychotherapy and memories of childhood sexual abuse: A cognitive perspective. *Applied Cognitive Psychology, 8*, 281–338.

54. Brewin, C.R. (2003). *Posttraumatic stress disorder: malady or myth?* New Haven: Yale University Press.

55. Pope, K.S. (1996). Memory, abuse, and science: Questioning claims about the false memory syndrome epidemic. *American Psychologist, 51*, 957–974.

56. Schooler, J.W., Bendiksen, M., & Ambadar, Z. (1997). Taking the middle line: Can we accommodate both fabricated and recovered memories of sexual abuse? In I.M. Conway (Ed.), *False and recovered memories* (pp. 251–292). Oxford: Oxford University Press.

57. Loftus, E.F. (1993). The reality of repressed memories. *Amer Psychol, 48*, 518–537.

58. Loftus, E.F., Polonsky, S., & Fullilove, M.T. (1994). Memories of childhood sexual abuse: Remembering and repressing. *Psychology of Women Quarterly, 18*, 67–84.

59. Elliott, D.M., & Briere, J. (1995). Posttraumatic stress associated with delayed recall of sexual abuse: A general population study. *Journal of Traumatic Stress, 8*, 629–648.

60. Chu, J.A. Frey, L.M., Ganzel, B.L., & Mathews, J.A. (1999). Memories of childhood abuse: Dissociation, amnesia, and corroboration. *American Journal of Psychiatry, 156*, 749–755.

61. Herman, J. (1992). *Trauma and recovery*. New York: Basic Books.

62. McCann, L., & Pearlman, A. (1990). Vicarious traumatization: A framework for understanding the psychological effects of working with victims. *Journal of Traumatic Stress, 3*, 131–149.

63. Figley, C.R. (1995). *Compassion fatigue: Secondary traumatic stress disorders from treating the traumatized*. New York: Brunner/Mazel.

64. Danieli, Y. (1984). Psychotherapists' participation in the conspiracy of silence about the Holocaust. *Psychoanalytic Psychology, 1*, 23–42.

65. Wilson, J., & Lindy, J. (1994). *Countertransference in the treatment of PTSD*. New York: Guilford Press.

66. Courtois, C.A. (1988). *Healing the incest wound: Adult survivors in therapy*. New York: W.W. Norton.

67. Yassen, J. (1993). Group work with clinicians who have a history of trauma. *NCP Clinical Newsletter, 3*:10–11.

68. Gould, M.,Greenberg, N. & Hetherton, J.(2007). Stigma and the military: Evaluation of a PTSD psychoeducational program. *Journal of Traumatic Stress, 20,* 505–515.

69. Olfaz, F., Hatipogiu, S., et al. (2008). Effectiveness of psychoeducation intervention on posttraumatic stress disorder and coping styles of earthquake survivors. *Journal of Clinical Nursing, 17,* 677–687.

70. Scholes, C., Turpin, G., & Mason, S. (2007) A randomized controlled trial to assess the effectiveness of providing self-help information to

people with symptoms of acute stress disorder following traumatic injury. *Behaviour Research and Therapy, 45,* 2527–2536.

71. Turpin, G., Downs, M., & Mason, S. (2005) Effectiveness of providing self-help information following acute traumatic injury: Randomized-controlled trial. *British Journal of Psychiatry, 187,* 76–82.

72. Adler,A., Bliese, P.D., McGurk, D., Hoge, C.W., & Castro, C.A. (2009) Battlemind debriefing and Battlemind training as early interventions with soldiers returning from Iraq: Randomization by platoon. *Journal of Consulting and Clinical Psychology, 77,* 928–940.

73. Cahill, S.P., Rothbaum, B.O., Resick, P., & Follette, V.M. (2009). Cognitive-behavioral therapy for adults.. In E.B. Foa, T.M. Keane, M.J. Friedman & J.A. Cohen (Eds.), *Effective treatments for PTSD: Practice Guidelines from the International Society for Traumatic Stress Studies* (2nd ed., pp. 139–222). New York: Guilford.

74. Foa, E.B., & Kozak, M.J. (1986). Emotional processing of fear: Exposure to corrective information. *Psychological Bulletin, 99,* 20–35.

75. Foa, E.B., Riggs, D.S., Massie, E.G., & Yarczower, M. (1995). The impact of fear activation and anger on the efficacy of exposure treatment for PTSD. *Behavior Therapy, 26,* 487–499.

76. Follette, V.M., & Ruzek, J.I. (2006). *Cognitive-behaviorial therapies for trauma* (2nd ed.). New York: Guilford.

77. Tarrier, N., Pilgrim, H., & Sommerfield, C., et al. (1999). A randomized trial of cognitive therapy and imaginal exposure in the treatment of chronic posttraumatic stress disorder. *J Consult and Clin Psychol, 67,* 13–18.

78. Rothbaum, B.O. (2009). Using virtual reality to help our patients in the real world.. *Depression and Anxiety, 26,* 209–211.

79. Lovell, K., Marks, I.M., Noshivarni, H., et al. (2001). Do cognitive and exposure treatments improve various PTSD symptoms differently? A randomized controlled trial. *Behav and Cognitive Psychotherapy, 29,* 107–112.

80. Resick, P., Nishith, P., Weaver, T., et al. (2002). A comparison of Cognitive Processing Therapy with Prolonged Exposure and a waiting condition for the treatment of chronic posttraumatic stress disorder in female rape victims. *J Consult and Clin Psychol, 70,* 867–879.

81. Hickling, E.J., & Blanchard, E.B. (1997). The private practice psychologist and manual-based treatments: Post-traumatic stress disorder secondary to motor vehicle accidents. *Behav Res Ther, 35,* 191–203.

82. Beck, A.T. (1976). *Cognitive therapy and the emotional disorders.* New York: International University Press.

83. Clark, D.M. (1986). A cognitive approach to panic. *Behaviour Research and Therapy, 24,* 461–470.

84. Marks, I., Lovell, K., Noshirvani, H., Livanou, M., & Thrasher, S. (1998). Treatment of post-traumatic stress disorder by exposure and/or cognitive restructuring: A controlled study. *Archives of General Psychiatry, 55,* 317–325.

85. Paunovic, N., & Ost, L. (2001). Cognitive-behavioral therapy vs. exposure therapy in the treatment of PTSD in refugees. *Behaviour Research and Therapy, 39,* 1183–1197.

86. Resick, P.A., & Schnicke, M.K. (1992). Cognitive processing therapy for sexual assault victims. *Journal of Consulting and Clinical Psychology, 60,* 748–756.

87. Resick, P.A., & Schnicke, M.K. (1993). *Cognitive processing therapy for rape victims: A treatment manual.* Newbury Park: Sage.

88. Kilpatrick, D.G., Veronen, L.J., & Resick, P.A. (1982). Psychological sequelae to rape: Assessment and treatment strategies. In D.M. Dolays & R.L. Meredith (Eds.), *Behavioral medicine: Assessment and treatment strategies* (pp. 473–497). New York: Plenum.

89. Resick, P.A., Jordan, C.G., Girelli, S.A., Hutter, C.K., & Marhoefer-Dvorak, S. (1988). A comparative victim study of behavioral group therapy for sexual assault victims. *Behavior Therapy, 19,* 385–401.

90. Foa, E.B., Dancu, C.V., Hembree, E.A., et al. (1999). A comparison of exposure therapy, stress inoculation training, and their combination for reducing posttraumatic stress disorder in female assault victims. *J Consult and Clin Psychology, 67,* 194–200.

91. Foa, E.B., Rothbaum, B.O., Riggs, D.S., et al. (1991). Treatment of posttraumatic stress disorder in rape victims: A comparison between cognitive-behavioral procedures and counseling. *J Consulting and Clin Psychology, 59,* 715–723.

92. Lange, A., van de Ven, J.P., Schrieken, B., & Emmelkamp, P.M.G. (2001). INTERAPY: Treatment of posttraumatic stress through the Internet. *Journal of Behavior Therapy & Experimental Psychiatry, 32,* 73–90.

93. Lange, A., Rietdijk, D., Judcovicova, M., van de Ven, J.P., Schrieken, B., & Emmelkamp, P.M.G. (2003). Interapy: A controlled randomized trial of the standard treatment of posttraumatic stress through the Internet. *Journal of Consulting & Clinical Psychology, 71,* 901–909.

94. Litz,B.T., Engel, C.C., Bryant, R.A., & Papa, A. (2007). A randomized controlled proof-of-concept trial of an Internet-based therapist-assisted, self-management treatment for posttraumatic stress disorder. *American Journal of Psychiatry, 164,* 1676–1683.

95. Hirai, M., & Clum, G.A. (2005) An Internet-based, self-change program for traumatic event related fear, distress and maladaptive coping. *Journal of Traumatic Stress, 18,* 631–636.

96. Krakow, B., Hollifield, M., Johnston, L., et al. (2001). Imagery rehearsal therapy for chronic nightmares in sexual assault survivors with posttraumatic stress disorder: A randomized controlled trial. *Journal of the American Medical Association, 286,* 537–545.

97. Forbes, D., Phleps, A., & McHugh, T. (2001). Treatment of combat-related nightmares using imagery rehearsal: A pilot study. *J Trauma Stress, 14,* 433–442.

98. Krakow, B., Sandoval, D., Schrader, R., et al. (2001). Treatment of chronic nightmares in adjudicated adolescent girls in a residential facility. *J Adolesc Health, 29,* 94–100.

99. Becker, C.B., & Zayfert, C. (2001). Integrating DBT-based techniques and concepts to facilitate exposure treatment for PTSD. *Cognitive & Behavioral Practice, 8,* 107–122.

100. Evans, K., Tyrer, P., et al. (1999). Manual-assisted cognitive-behaviour therapy (MACT): A randomized controlled trial of a brief intervention with bibliotherapy in the treatment of recurrent deliberate self-harm. *Psychological Medicine, 29,* 19–25.

101. Hawton, K., Townsend, E., et al. (2000). *Psychosocial versus pharmacological treatments for deliberate self-harm.* Cochrane Database Syst Rev. CD001764.

102. Spates, C.R., Koch, E., Cusak, K., Pagato, S., & Waller, S. (2009). Eye movement desentization and reprocessing. In E.B. Foa, T.M. Keane,

M.J. Friedman, & J.A. Cohen (Eds.), *Effective treatments for PTSD: Practice guidelines from the International Society for Traumatic Stress Studies* (2nd ed., pp. 279–305). New York: Guilford.

103. Shapiro, F. (1989). Eye movement desensitization: A new treatment for post-traumatic stress disorder. *Journal of Behavior Therapy and Experimental Psychiatry, 20*, 211–217.

104. Shapiro, F. (1995). *Eye movement desensitization and reprocessing: Basic principles, protocols, and procedures.* New York: Guilford.

105. McNally, R.J. (1999). Research on eye movement desensitization and reprocessing (EMDR) as a treatment for PTSD. *PTSD Research Quarterly, 10*, 1–7.

106. Hyer, L. & Brandsma, J.M. (1997). EMDR minus eye movements equals good psychotherapy. *Journal of Traumatic Stress, 10*, 515–522.

107. Ironson, G., Freund, B., Strauss, J.L., et al. (2002). Comparison of two treatments for traumatic stress: A community-based study of EMDR and prolonged exposure. *J Clin Psychol, 58*, 113–128.

108. Jensen, J.A. (1994). An investigation of Eye Movement Desensitization and Reprocessing (EMD/R) as a treatment for Posttraumatic Stress Disorder (PTSD) symptoms of Vietnam combat veterans. *Behav Therapy, 25*, 311–325.

109. Taylor, S., Thordurson, D.S., Maxfield, I., Federoff, I.C., Lovell, K., & Ogrodniczuk, J. (2003). Comparative efficacy, speed and adverse effects of three PTSD treatments: Exposure therapy, EMDR and relaxation training. *Journal of Consulting and Clinical Psychology, 71*, 330–338.

110. van der Kolk, B.A., Spinazzola, J., Blaustein, M.E., Hopper, J.W., Hopper, E.K., Korn, D.L., et al. (2007). A randomized clinical trial of eye movement desensitization and reprocessing EMDR, fluoxetine and pill placebo in the treatment of posttraumatic stress disorder: Treatment effects and long-term maintenance. *Journal of Clinical Psychiatry, 68,* 37–46.

111. Rothbaum, B.O., Astrin, M.C., & Marsteller, F. (2005). Prolonged exposure versus eye movement desensitization and reprocessing (EMDR) for PTSD rape victims. *Journal of Traumatic Stress, 18,* 607–616.

112. Power, K., McGoldrick, T., Brown, K. Buchanan, R., Sharp, D., Swanson, V., et al. (2002). A controlled comparison of eye movement desensitization and reprocessing versus exposure plus cognitive restructuring versus waiting list in the treatment of posttraumatic stress disorder. *Clinical Psychology and Psychotherapy, 9,* 299–318.

113. Lee, C., Gavriel, H., Drummond, P., Richards, J., & Greenwald, R. (2002). Treatment of PTSD; Stress inoculation training with prolonged exposure compared to EMDR. *Journal of Clinical Psychology, 58,* 1071–1089.

114. Devilly, G.J., & Spence, S.H. (1999). The relative efficacy and treatment distress of EMDR and a cognitive behavioral trauma treatment protocol in the amelioration of post traumatic stress disorder. *Journal of Anxiety Disorders, 13*, 131–158.

115. Foa, E., & Meadows, E. (1997). Psychosocial treatments for posttraumatic stress disorder: A critical review. *Ann Rev Psychol, 48*, 449–480.

116. Davidson, P.R., & Parker, K.C. (2001). Eye movement desensitization and reprocessing (EMDR): A meta-analysis. *J Consult & Clin Psychol, 69*, 305–316.

117. Seidler, G.H., & Wagner, F.E. (2006) Comparing the efficacy of EMDR and trauma-focused cognitive behavioral therapy in the treatment of PTSD: A meta-analytic study. *Psychological Medicine, 6,* 1–8.

118. Van Etten, M.L., & Taylor, S. (1998). Comparative efficacy of treatments for posttraumatic stress disorder: A meta-analysis. *Clinical Psychology and Psychotherapy, 5,* 126–144.

119. Bradley, R., Green, J., Russ, E., Dutra, L., & Westen, D. (2005). A multidimensional meta-analysis of psychotherapy for PTSD. *American Journal of Psychiatry, 162,* 214–227.

120. Kudler, H., Krupnick, J., Blank, A.S., Herman, J.L., & Horowitz, M.J. (2009). Psychodynamic therapy for adults. In E.B. Foa, T.M. Keane, M.J. Friedman , & J.A. Cohen (Eds.), *Practice Guidelines for PTSD* (2nd ed.) (pp. 346–369). New York: Guilford.

121. Horowitz, M.J. (1974). Stress response syndromes: Character style and dynamic psychotherapy. *Archives of General Psychiatry, 31,* 768–781.

122. Krystal, H. (1988). *Integration and self healing.* Hillsdale, NJ: The Analytic Press.

123. Lindy, J. (1996). Psychoanalytic psychotherapy of post-traumatic stress disorder. In B. van der Kolk, A. McFarlane, & L. Weisaeth (Eds.), *Traumatic stress* (pp. 525–536). New York: Guilford Press.

124. Marmar, C. & Freeman, M. (1988). Brief dynamic psychotherapy for post-traumatic stress disorders: Management of narcissistic regression. *Journal of Traumatic Stress, 1,* 323–337.

125. Brom, D., Kleber, R.J., & Defares, P.B. (1989). Brief psychotherapy for post-traumatic stress disorders. *Journal of Consulting and Clinical Psychology, 57,* 607–612.

126. Courtois, C.A. (1999) *Recollections of sexual abuse: Treatment principles and guidelines.* New York, Norton.

127. Roth, S., & Bateson, R. (1997). *Naming the shadows: A new approach to individual and group psychotherapy for adult survivors of childhood incest.* New York: Free Press.

128. Shengold, L. (1989). *Soul murder: The effects of childhood abuse and deprivation.* New Haven, CT: Yale University Press.

129. Shea, M.T., McDevitt-Murphy, M., Ready, D.J., & Schnurr, P.P. (2009). Group therapy. In E.B. Foa, T.M. Keane, M.J. Friedman, & J.A. Cohen (Eds.), *Effective Treatments for PTSD: Practice Guidelines from the International Society for Traumatic Stress Studies* (2nd ed., pp. 306–326). New York: Guilford.

130. Yalom, I.D. (1975). The theory and practice of group psychotherapy. New York: Basic Books.

131. Roth, S.H., Dye, E., & Lebowitz, L. (1988). Group therapy for sexual assault victims. *Psychotherapy, 25,* 82–93.

132. Foy, D.W., Ruzek, J.I., Glynn, S.M., Riney, S.A., & Gusman, F.D. (1997). Trauma focus group therapy for combat-related PTSD. *In Session: Psychotherapy in Practice, 3,* 59–73.

133. Ready, D.J., Thomas, K.R., Worley, V., Backscheider, A.G., Harvey, L.A., Baltzell, D., et al. (2008). A field test of group based exposure therapy with 102 veterans with war-related posttraumatic stress disorder. *Journal of Traumatic Stress, 21,* 150–157.

134. Schnurr, P.P., Friedman, M.J., Foy, D.W., Shea, M.T., Hsieh, F.Y., Lavori, P.W.,et al. (2003). Randomized trial of trauma-focused group

therapy for posttraumatic stress disorder. *Archives of General Psychiatry, 60,* 481–489.

135. Riggs, D.S. (2000). Marital and family therapy. In E.B. Foa, T.M. Keane, & M.J. Friedman (Eds.), *Practice Guidelines for PTSD* (pp. 280–301). New York: Guilford.

136. Waysman, M., Mikulincer, M., & Solomon, Z., et al. (1993). Secondary traumatization among wives of posttraumatic combat veterans: A family typology. *Journal of Family Psychology, 7,* 104–118.

137. Figley, C.R. (1989). *Helping traumatized families.* San Francisco: Jossey-Bass.

138. Harris, C.J. (1991). A family crisis-intervention model for the treatment of post-traumatic stress reaction. *Journal of Traumatic Stress, 4,* 195–207.

139. Rosenheck, R., & Thompson, J. (1986). "Detoxification" of Vietnam war trauma: A combined family-individual approach. *Family Process, 25,* 559–570.

140. Williams, C.M., & Williams, T. (1980). Family therapy for Vietnam veterans. In T. Williams (Ed.), *Post-traumatic stress disorder of the Vietnam veteran.* Cincinnati, OH: Disabled American Veterans.

141. Mueser, K.T., & Glynn, S.M. (1995). *Behavioral family therapy for psychiatric disorders.* Needham Heights, MA: Allyn & Bacon.

142. Monson, C.M., Schnurr, P.P., Stevens, S.P., & Guthrie, K.A. (2004) Cognitive-behavioral couples treatment for posttraumatic stress disorder: Initial findings. *Journal of Traumatic Stress, 17,* 341–344.

143. Monson, C.M., Schnurr, P.P., & Stevens, S.P. (2005). Cognitive-behavioral couples treatment for posttraumatic stress disorder. In T.A. Corales (Ed.), *Focus on posttraumatic stress disorder* (pp.245–274). Hauppauge, NY: Nova Science.

144. Devilly, G.J. (2002). The psychological effects of a lifestyle management course on war veterans and their spouses. *Journal of Clinical Psychology, 58,* 1119–1134.

145. Cardena, E., Maldonado, J., van der Hart, O., & Spiegel, D. (2000). Hypnosis. In E.B. Foa, T.M. Keane, & M.J. Friedman (Eds.), *Practice Guidelines for PTSD* (pp. 247–279). New York: Guilford.

146. Bryant, R.A., Moulds, M.L., Guthrie, R.M. & Nixon, R.D.V. (2005). The additive benefit of hypnosis and cognitive-behavioral therapy in treating acute stress disorder. *Journal of Consulting and Clinical Psychology, 73,* 334–340.

147. Mueser, K.T., Salyers, M.P., Rosenberg, S.D., Ford, J.D., Fox, L., & Carty, P. (2001). Psychometric evaluation of trauma and posttraumatic stress disorder assessments in persons with severe mental illness. *Psychological Assessment, 13,* 110–117.

148. Penk, W. Binus, G., & Herz, L. et al. (2000). Psychosocial rehabilitation techniques. In E.B. Foa, T.M. Keane, & M.J. Friedman (Eds.), *Practice Guidelines for PTSD* (pp 224–246). New York: Guilford.

149. Pynoos, R.S. (1993). Traumatic stress and developmental psychopathology in children and adolescents. In J.M. Oldham, M.B. Riba, & A. Tasman (Eds.), *Review of Psychiatry, Volume 12* (pp. 205–238). Washington, DC: American Psychiatric Press.

150. Fairbank, J.A., Putnam, F.W., & Harris, W.W. (2007) The prevalence and impact of child traumatic stress. In M.J. Friedman, T.M. Keane, & P.A. Resick (Eds.), *Handbook of PTSD: Science and practice* (pp. 229–251). New York: Guilford.

151. Pynoos, R.S., Steinberg, A.M., & Wraith, R. (1995). A developmental model of childhood traumatic stress. In D. Cicchetti & D. Cohen (Eds.), *Manual of developmental psychology, vol 2: Risk, disorder, and adaptation.* New York: John Wiley.

152. Terr, L.C. (1989). Treating psychic trauma in children. *Journal of Traumatic Stress, 2,* 3–19.

153. Putnam, F.W. (1997). *Dissociation in children and adolescents: A developmental perspective.* New York: Guilford.

154. Herman, J.L., Perry, J.C., & van der Kolk, B.A. (1989). Childhood trauma in borderline personality disorder. *American Journal of Psychiatry, 146,* 490–495.

155. Lyons, J.A. (1987). Posttraumatic stress disorder in children and adolescents: A review of the literature. *Dev Behav Pediatr, 8,* 349–356.

156. Cohen, J.A., Mannarino, A.P., Deblinger, E., & Berliner, L. (2009). Cognitive-behavioral therapy for children and adolescents. In E.B. Foa, T.M. Keane, M.J. Friedman, & J.A. Cohen (Eds.), *Effective treatments for PTSD: Practice guidelines from the International Society for Traumatic Stress Studies* (2nd ed., pp. 223–244). New York: Guilford.

157. Smith P., Yule, W., Perrin, S., Tranah, T., Dalgleish, T. & Clark, D. (2007). Cognitive behavior therapy for PTSD in children and adolescents: A preliminary randomized controlled trial. *Journal of the American Academy of Child and Adolescent Psychiatry, 46,* 1051–1061.

158. Najavits, L.M., Gallop, R.J., & Weiss, R.D. (2006). Seeking Safety therapy for adolescent girls with PTSD and substance use disorder: A randomized controlled trial. *Journal of Behavioral Health Services Research, 33,* 453–463.

159. Jaycox, L.H., Stein, B.D., & Amaya-Jackson, L. (2009). School-based treatments for children and adolescents. In E.B. Foa, T.M. Keane, M.J. Friedman, & J.A. Cohen (Eds.), *Effective treatments for PTSD: Practice guidelines from the International Society for Traumatic Stress Studies* (2nd ed., pp. 327–345). New York: Guilford.

160. Jaycox, L.H. (2005) *Cognitive-behavioral interventions for trauma in schools.* Longmont, CO: Sopris West Educational Services.

161. Amaya-Jackson, L., Reynolds, V., Murray, M.C., McCarthy, G., Nelson, A., Cherney, M.S., et al. (2003). Cognitive behavioral treatment for pediatric posttraumatic stress disorder: Protocol and application in school and community settings. *Cognitive Behavioral Practice, 10,* 204–213.

162. Goenjian, A.K., Walling, D., Steinberg, A.M., Karayan, I., Najarian, L.M., & Pynoos, R.S. (2005). A prospective study of posttraumatic stress and depressive reactions among treated and untreated adolescents 5 years after a catastrophic disaster. *American Journal of Psychiatry, 162,* 2302–2308.

163. Lieberman, A.F., Ippen, C.G., & Marans, S.R. (2009). Psychodynamic therapy for child trauma. In E.B. Foa, T.M. Keane, M.J. Friedman, & J.A. Cohen (Eds.), *Effective treatments for PTSD: Practice guidelines from the International Society for Traumatic Stress Studies* (2nd ed., pp. 370–387). New York: Guilford.

164. Dozier, M., Peloso, E., Linheim, O., Gordon, M.K., Manni, M., Sepulveda, S., et al. (2006). Preliminary evidence from a randomized clinical trial: Intervention effects on foster children's behavioral and biological regulation. *Journal of Social Issues, 62,* 767–785.

165. Trowell, J., Kolvin, I., Werramanthri, T., Sadowski, H., Berelowitz, M., Glasser, D., et al. (2002). Psychotherapy for sexually abused girls: Psychopathological outcome findings and patterns. *British Journal of Psychiatry, 180,* 234–247.

166. Goodman, R.F., Chapman, L.M., & Gantt, L. (2009) Creative art therapies for children. In E.B. Foa, T.M. Keane, M.J. Friedman, & J.A. Cohen (Eds.), *Effective treatments for PTSD: Practice guidelines from the International Society for Traumatic Stress Studies* (2nd ed., pp. 491–507). New York: Guilford.

167. Chapman, L., Morabito, D., Ladakakos, C., Schreier, H., & Knudson, M. (2001). The effectiveness of art therapy interventions in reducing post-traumatic stress disorder (PTSD) symptoms in pediatric trauma patients. *Art Therapy: Journal of the American Art therapy Association, 18,* 100–104.

168. Cannon, W.B. (1932). *The wisdom of the body.* New York: Norton.

169. Neumeister, A., Henry, S., & Krystal, J.H. (2007). Neurocircuitry and neuroplasticity. In M.J. Friedman, T.M. Keane, & P.A. Resick (Eds). *Handbook of PTSD: Science and practice* (pp. 166–189). New York: Guilford.

170. Southwick, S.M., Davis, L.L., Aikins, D.E., Rassmusson, A, Barron J., & Morgan, C.A. (2007). Neurobiological alterations associated with PTSD. In M.J. Friedman, T.M. Keane, P.A. Resick (Eds.), *Handbook of PTSD: Science and practice* (pp. 190–206). New York: Guilford.

171. Selye, H. (1946). The general adaptation syndrome and the diseases of adaptation. *J Clin Endocrinol, 6*: 117–230.

172. Chrousos, G.P., & Gold, P.W. (1992). The concepts of stress and stress system disorders: Overview of physical and behavioral homeostasis. *JAMA, 267,* 1244–1252.

173. Malloy, P., Fairbank, J., & Keane, T. (1983). Validation of a multimethod assessment of posttraumatic stress disorder in Vietnam veterans. *J Consult Clin Psychol, 51,* 488–493.

174. Pitman, R., Orr, S., Forgue, D., et al. (1987). Psychophysiologic assessment of posttraumatic stress disorder imagery in Vietnam combat veterans. *Arch Gen Psychiatry, 44,* 970–975.

175. Southwick, S.M., Krystal, J.H., Morgan, A.C., et al. (1993). Abnormal noradrenergic function in post-traumatic stress disorder. *Arch Gen Psychiatry, 50,* 266–274 .

176. Bremner, J.D., Licinio, J., Darnell, A., et al. (1997). Elevated CRF corticotropin-releasing factor concentrations in post-traumatic stress disorder. *Am J Psychiatry 154,* 624–629.

177. Yehuda R, & McFarlane A.C. (1995). Conflict between current knowledge about posttraumatic stress disorder and its original conceptual basis. *Am J Psychiatry, 152,* 1705–1713.

178. Friedman, M.J., & Davidson, J.R.T. (2007). Pharmacotherapy. In M.J. Friedman, T.M. Keane, & P.A. Resick (Eds.), *Handbook of PTSD: Science and practice* (pp. 376–405). New York: Guilford.

179. Friedman, M.J., Davidson, J.R.T. & Stein, D.S. (2009) Pharmacotherapy for adults. In E.B. Foa, T.M. Keane, M.J. Friedman & J.A. Cohen (Eds.), *Effective treatments for PTSD: Practice guidelines from the International Society for Traumatic Stress Studies* (pp. 245–268). New York: Guilford.

180. Brady, K., Pearlstein, T., Asnis, G.M., et al. (2000). Efficacy and safety of sertraline treatment of posttraumatic stress disorder. *JAMA, 283,* 1837–1844.

181. Davidson, J.R.T., Rothbaum, B.O., van der Kolk, B.A., et al. (2001). Multicenter, double-blind comparison of sertraline and placebo in the treatment of posttraumatic stress disorder. *Archives of General Psychiatry, 58*, 485–492.

182. Marshall, R.D., Beebe, K.L., Oldham, M., & Zaninelli, R. (2001). Efficacy and safety of paroxetine treatment for chronic PTSD: A fixed-dose-placebo-controlled study. *American Journal of Psychiatry, 158*, 1982–1988.

183. Tucker, P., Zaninelli, R., Yehuda, R., Ruggiero, L., Dillingham, K., & Pitts, C.D. (2001). Paroxetine in the treatment of chronic post-traumatic stress disorder: Results of a placebo-controlled, flexible-dosage trial. *Journal of Clinical Psychiatry, 62*, 860–868.

184. Davidson, J.R.T., Baldwin, D.V., Stein, D.J., Kuper, E., Benattia, I., Ahmen, S., et al. (2006). Treatment of posttraumatic stress disorder with venlafaxine extended release: A six month randomized controlled trial. *Archives of General Psychiatry, 63*, 1158–1165.

185. Davidson, J.R.T., Rothbaum, B.O., Tucker, P.M., Asnis, G.M., Benattia, I., & Musgnung, J.J. (2006). Venlafaxine extended release in posttraumatic stress disorder: A sertraline- and placebo-controlled study. *Journal of Clinical Psychopharmacology, 26*, 259–267.

186. Davis, M., Ressler, K., Rothbaum, B.O., & Richardson, R. (2006). Effects of D-cycloserine on extinction: Translation from preclinical to clinical work. *Biological Psychiatry, 60,* 369–375.

187. Rothbaum, B.O. (2008). Critical parameters for D-cycloserine enhancement of cognitive-behaviorial therapy for obsessive-compulsive disorder. *American Journal of Psychiatry, 165*(3), 293–296.

188. Martenyi, F., Brown, E.B., Zhang, H., Prakash, A., & Koke, S.C. (2002). Fluoxetine versus placebo in posttraumatic stress disorder. *Journal of Clinical Psychiatry, 63*, 199–206.

189. Seedat, S., Lockhat, R., Kaminer, D., Zungu-Dirwayi, N., & Stein, D.J. (2001). An open trial of citalopram in adolescents with post-traumatic stress disorder. *Int Clin Psychopharmacol, 16*, 21–25.

190. Whittington, C. J., Kendall, R., Fonagy, P., Cottrell, D., Cotgrove, A., & Boddington, E. (2004). Selective serotonin reuptake inhibitors in childhood depression: Systematic review of published versus unpublished data. *The Lancet, 363*, 1341–45.

191. U.S. Food and Drug Administration. (2004). *FDA Talk Paper: FDA issues public health advisory on cautions for use of antidepressants in adults and children* (T04-08, March 22, 2004). Retrieved from: http://www.fda.gov.

192. Lonborg, P.D., Hegel, M.T., Goldstein, S., Goldstein, D., Himmelhoch, J.M., Maddock, R., et al. (2001). Sertraline treatment of posttraumatic stress disorder: Results of weeks of open-label continuation treatment. *J Clin Psychiatry, 62*, 325–331.

193. Rothbaum, B.O., Cahill, S.P., Foa, E.B., Davidson, J.R.T., Compton, J.S., Connor, K.M., et al. (2006). Augmentation of sertraline with prolonged exposure in the treatment of posttraumatic stress disorder. *Journal of Traumatic Stress, 19*, 625–638.

194. DeMartino, R., Mollica, R.F., & Wilk, V. (1995). Monoamine oxidase inhibitors in posttraumatic stress disorder. *J Nerv Ment Dis, 183*, 510–515.

195. Southwick, S.M., Yehuda, R., Giller, E.L., et al. (1994). Use of tricyclics and monoamine oxidase inhibitors in the treatment of PTSD: A

quantitative review. In M.M. Murburg (Ed.), *Catecholamine function in post-traumatic stress disorder: Emerging concepts* (pp. 293–305). Washington, DC: American Psychiatry Press.

196. Raskind, M.A., Peskind, E.R., Hoff, D.J., Hart, K.L., Holmes, H.A., Warren, D., et al. (2007). A parallel group placebo controlled study of prazosin for trauma nightmares and sleep disturbances in combat veterans with post-traumatic stress disorder. *Biological Psychiatry, 61*, 928–934.

197. Raskind, M.A., Peskind, E.R., Kanter, E.D., Petrie, E.C., Radant, A.D., Thompson, C.E., et al. (2003). Reduction of nightmares and other PTSD symptoms in combat veterans by prazosin: A placebo-controlled study. *American Journal of Psychiatry, 160*, 371–373.

198. Famularo, R., Kinscherff, R., & Fenton, T. (1988). Propranolol treatment for childhood posttraumatic stress disorder, acute type. *Am J Dis Child, 142*, 1244–1247.

199. Davis, L.L., Ward, C., Rasmusson, A., Newell, J.M., Frazier, E., & Southwick, S.M. (2008). A placebo-controlled trial of guanfacine for the treatment of posttraumatic stress disorder in veterans. *Psychopharmacology Bulletin 41*(1), 8–18.

200. Neylan, T.C., Lenoci, M.A., Samuelson, K.W., Metzler, T.J., Henn-Haase, C., Hierholzer, R.W., et al. (2006). No improvement of posttraumatic stress disorder symptoms with guanfacine treatment. *American Journal of Psychiatry, 163*, 2186–2188.

201. Kinzie, J.D., & Friedman, M.J. (2004). Psychopharmacology for refugee and asylum seeker patients. In J. P. Wilson & B. Drozdek (Eds.), *Broken spirits: The treatment of asylum seekers and refugees with PTSD* (pp. 579–600). New York: Brunner-Routledge Press.

202. Post, R.M., Weiss, S.R.B., & Smith, M.A. (1995). Sensitization and kindling: Implications for the evolving neural substrate of PTSD. In M.J. Friedman, D.S. Charney, & A.Y. Deutch (Eds), *Neurobiological and clinical consequences of stress: From normal adaptation to PTSD* (pp. 203–224). Philadelphia: Lippincott-Raven Press.

203. Davidson, J.R.T., Brady, K.T., Mellman, T.A., Stein, M.B., & Pollack, M.H. (2007). The efficacy and tolerability of tiagabine in adult patients with posttraumatic stress disorder. *Journal of Clinical Psychopharmacology, 27*, 85–88.

204. Davis, L.L., Davidson, J.R.T., Ward, L.C., Bartolucci, A.A., Bowden, C., & Petty, F. (2008). Divalproex in the treatment of posttraumatic stress disorder: A randomized, double-blind, placebo-controlled trial in a veteran population. *Journal of Clinical Psychopharmacology, 28*, 84–88.

205. Tucker, P.M., Trautman, R.P., Wyatt, D.B., Thompson, J., Wu, S.-C., Capece, J. A., et al. (2007). Efficacy and safety of topiramate monotherapy in civilian posttraumatic stress disorder: A randomized, double-blind, placebo-controlled study. *Journal of Clinical Psychiatry, 68*(2), 201–206.

206. Braun, P., Greenberg, D., Dasberg, H. et al. (1990). Core symptoms of posttraumatic stress disorder unimproved by alprazolam treatment. *J Clin Psychiatry 51*, 236–238.

207. Bouton, M.E., Kenney, F.A., & Rosengard, C. (1990). State-dependent fear extinction with two benzodiazepine tranquilizers. *Behavioral Neuroscience, 104*(1), 44–55.

208. van Minnen, A., Arntz, A., & Keijsers, G.P.J. (2002). Prolonged exposure in patients with chronic PTSD: Predictors of treatment

outcome and dropout. *Behaviour Research and Therapy, 40*(4), 439–457.

209. Monnelly, E.P., Ciraulo, D.A., Knapp, C., & Keane, T. (1999). Low dose risperidone as adjunctive therapy for irritable aggression in posttraumatic stress disorder. *J Clinical Psychopharmacology, 19*, 377–378.

210. Bartzokis, G., Lu, P.H., Turner, J., Mintz, J., & Saunders, C.S. (2005). Adjunctive risperidone in the treatment of chronic combat-related posttraumatic stress disorder. *Biological Psychiatry, 57*, 474–479.

211. Hamner, M.B., Faldowski, R.A., Ulmer, H.G., Frueh, B.C., Huber, M.G., & Arana, G.W. (2003). Adjunctive risperidone treatment in post-traumatic stress disorder: A preliminary controlled trial of effects on comorbid psychotic symptoms. *International Clinical Psychopharmacology, 18*, 1–8.

212. Reich, D.B., Winternitz, S., Hennen, J., Watts, T., & Stanculescu, C. (2004). A preliminary study of risperidone in the treatment of posttraumatic stress disorder related to childhood abuse in women. *Journal of Clinical Psychiatry, 65*, 1601–1606.

213. Sokolski, K.N., Denson, T.F., Lee, R.T., & Reist, C. (2003). Quetiapine for treatment of refractory symptoms of combat-related post-traumatic stress disorder. *Military Medicine, 168*, 486–489.

214. Stein, M.B., Kline, N.A., & Matloff, J.L. (2002). Adjunctive olanzapine for SSRI-resistant combat-related PTSD: A double-blind, placebo-controlled study. *American Journal of Psychiatry, 159*, 1777–1779.

215. Norris, F., Friedman, M., Watson, P., Byrne, C., Diaz, E., & Kaniasty, K. (2002). 60,000 disaster victims speak, Part I: An empirical review of the empirical literature, 1981–2001. *Psychiatry, 65*, 207–239.

216. Norris, F., Friedman, M., & Watson, P. (2002). 60,000 disaster victims speak, Part II: Summary and implications of the disaster mental health research. *Psychiatry, 65*, 240–260.

217. Norris, F.H., Murphy, A.D., Baker, C.K., & Perilla, J.L. (2003). Severity, timing and duration of reactions to trauma in the population: An example from Mexico. *Biol Psychiatry, 53*, 769–778.

218. Schuster, M., Bradley, D., Stein, M., Jaycox, L.H., Collins, R.L., Marshall, G.N., et al. (2001). A national survey of stress reactions after the September 11, 2001, terrorist attacks. *New England Journal of Medicine, 345*, 1507–1512.

219. Galea, S., Ahern, J., Resnick, H.S., Kilpatrick, D.G., Bucuvalas, M.J., Gold, J., et al. (2002). Psychological sequelae of the September 11 terrorist attacks in New York City. *New England Journal of Medicine, 346*, 982–987.

220. Tanielian,T.L., Jaycox, L., & Rand Corporation (Eds.) (2008). *Invisible wounds of war: Psychological and cognitive injuries, their consequences, and services to assist recovery.* Santa Monica, CA: RAND.

221. Gawande, A. (2004). Casualties of war—Military care for the wounded from Iraq and Afghanistan. *New England Journal of Medicine, 351*, 2471–2475.

222. Friedman, M.J. (2005). Veterans mental health in the wake of war. *New England Journal of Medicine, 352*, 1287–1290.

223. Stein, M.B., & McAllister, T.W. (2009). Exploring the convergency of posttraumatic stress disorder and mild traumatic brain injury. *American Journal of Psychiatry,166*, 768–776.

224. Litz, B.T., & Maguen, S. (2007). Early intervention for trauma. In M.J. Friedman, T.M. Keane, & P.A. Resick (Eds.), *Handbook of PTSD: Science and practice* (pp. 306–329). New York: Guilford.

225. Watson, P.J. (2007) Early intervention for trauma-related problems following mass trauma. In R.J. Ursano, C.S. Fullerton, L. Weisaeth, & B. Raphael (Eds.), *Textbook of disaster psychiatry* (pp. 121–139). Cambridge, UK: Cambridge University Press.

226. Friedman, M.J. (2005). Towards a public mental health approach for survivors of bioterrorism. In Y. Danieli & D. Brom (Eds.), *The trauma of terror: Sharing knowledge and shared care* (pp. 527–540). New York: Guilford.

227. Naturale, A.J. (in press). Mental health outreach strategies: An experiential description of the outreach methodologies utilized in the New York 9/11 disaster response. In E.C. Ritchie, M.J. Friedman, & P.J. Watson (Eds.), *Psychological and public health interventions following mass violence and disasters*. New York: Guilford.

228. Solomon, Z., & Benbenishty, R. (1986). The role of proximity, immediacy, and expectancy in frontline treatment of combat stress reaction among Israelis in the Lebanon War. *American Journal of Psychiatry, 143*, 613–617.

229. National Institute of Mental Health (2002). *Mental health and mass violence: Evidence-based early intervention for victims/survivors of mass violence: A workshop to reach consensus on best practices*. Washington, DC: U.S. Government Printing Office.

230. Bisson, J.I., McFarlane, A.C., Ruzek, J.I., Watson, P.J., & Rose, S. (2009). Psychological debriefing for adults. In E.B. Foa, T.M. Keane, M.J. Friedman, & J.A. Cohen (Eds.), *Effective treatments for PTSD: Practice guidelines from the International Society for Traumatic Stress Studies* (2nd ed., pp. 83–105). New York: Guilford.

231. Nash, W.P., Steenkamp, M., Conoscenti, L., & Litz, B.T. (in press). The stress continuum model: A military organizational approach to resilience and recovery. In S.M. Southwick, B.T. Litz, D.S. Charney, & M.J. Friedman (Eds.), *Comprehensive textbook of resilience*. Cambridge, UK: Cambridge University Press.

232. Mitchell, J.T. (1983). When disaster strikes . . . *Journal of Emergency Medical Services, 8*, 36–39.

233. Dyregrov, A. (1989). Caring for helpers in disaster situations: Psychological debriefing. *Disaster Management, 2*, 25–30.

234. Rose, S., Bisson, J., & Wessely, S. (2002). Psychological debriefing for preventing posttraumatic stress disorder (PTSD) (Cochrane review). In *The Cochrane Library,* Issue 2. Oxford, UK: Update Software.

235. Bisson, J.I., Jenkins, P.L., Alexander, J., & Bannister, C. (1997). Randomized controlled trial of psychological debriefing for victims of acute burn trauma. *Br J Psychiatry, 171*, 78–81.

236. Mayou, R.A., Ehlers, A., & Hobbs, M. (2000). A three-year follow-up of psychological debriefing for road traffic accident victims. *Br J Psychiatry, 176*, 589–593.

237. Ehlers, A., & Clark, D.M. (2003). Early psychological interventions for adult survivors of trauma: A review. *Biol Psychiatry, 53*, 817–826.

238. Foa, E.B., & Cahill, S.P. (2001). Psychological therapies: Emotional processing. In N.J. Smelser & P.B. Bates (Eds.), *International encyclopedia of the social and behavioral sciences* (pp. 12363–12369). Oxford: Elsevier.

239. Bryant, R.A. (2003). Early predictors of posttraumatic stress disorder. *Biol Psychiatry, 53,* 789–795.

240. McNally, R.J. (2003). Psychological mechanisms in acute response to trauma. *Biol Psychiatry, 53,* 779–788.

241. Shalev, A.Y., Sahar, T., Freedman, S., Peri, T., Glick, N., Brandes, D., et al. (1998). A prospective study of heart rate response following trauma and subsequent development of posttraumatic stress disorder. *Arch Gen Psychiatry, 55,* 553–559.

242. Bryant, R.A., Harvey, A.G., Guthrie, R.M., & Moulds, M.L. (2000). A prospective study of psychophysiological arousal, acute stress disorder and posttraumatic stress disorder. *J Abnorm Psychol, 109,* 341–344.

243. Morgan, C.A., Krystal, J.H., & Southwick, S.M. (2003). Toward early pharmacologic post-traumatic stress intervention. *Biol Psychiatry, 53,* 834–843.

244. Ehlers, A., & Steil, R. (1995). *An experimental study of intrusive memories.* Paper presented at the World Congress of Behavioural and Cognitive Therapies; Copenhagen, Denmark.

245. Classen, C., Koopman, C., Hales, R., & Spiegel, D. (1998). Acute stress disorder as a predictor of posttraumatic stress symptoms. *Am J Psychiatry, 155,* 620–624.

246. Eriksson, N.G., & Lundin, T. (1996). Early traumatic stress reactions among Swedish survivors of the m/s *Estonia* disaster. *Br J Psychiatry, 169,* 713–716.

247. Staab, J.P., Grieger, T.A., Fullerton, C.S., & Ursano, R.J. (1996). Acute stress disorder, subsequent posttraumatic stress disorder and depression after a series of typhoons. *Anxiety, 2,* 219–225.

248. Bryant, R.A., & Harvey, A.G. (1998). Relationship between acute stress disorder and posttraumatic stress disorder following mild traumatic brain injury. *Am J Psychiatry, 155,* 625–629.

249. Daviss, W.B., Racusin, R., Fleischer, A., Mooney, D., Ford, J.D., & McHugo, G.J. (2000). Acute stress disorder symptomatology during hospitalization for pediatric injury. *J Am Acad Child Adolesc Psychiatry 39,* 569–575.

250. Bryant, R.A. (2003). Early predictors of posttraumatic stress disorder. *Biological Psychiatry, 53,* 789–795.

251. Bryant, R.A., Harvey, A.G., Dang, S., & Sackville, T. (1998). Assessing acute stress disorder: Psychometric properties of a structured clinical interview. *Psychological Assessment, 10,* 215–220.

252. Bryant, R.A., Moulds, M., & Guthrie, R. (2000). Acute stress disorder scale: A self-report measure of acute stress disorder. *Psychological Assessment, 12,* 61–68.

253. Cardena, E., Koopman, C., Classen, C., Waelde, L.C., & Spiegel, D. (2000). Psychometric properties of the Stanford Acute Stress Reaction Questionnaire: A valid and reliable measure of acute stress. *Journal of Traumatic Stress, 13,* 719–734.

254. Bryant R.A., Harvey A.G., & Dang S.T., et al. (1998). Treatment of acute stress disorder: A comparison of cognitive-behavioral therapy and supportive counseling. *J Consult Clin Psychol, 66,* 862–866.

255. Bryant R.A., Sackville T., Dang S.T., et al. (1999). Treating acute stress disorder: An evaluation of cognitive behavior therapy and supportive counseling techniques. *Am J Psychiatry, 156,* 1780–1786.

256. Bryant, R.A., Moulds, M.L., & Nixon, R.D.V. (2003). Cognitive therapy of acute stress disorder: A four-year follow-up. *Behav Res Ther, 41*, 489–494.

257. Foa, E.B., Hearst-Ikeda, D., & Perry, K.J. (1995). Evaluation of a brief cognitive-behavioral program for the prevention of chronic PTSD in recent assault victims. *J Consult Clin Psychol, 63*, 948–955.

258. Pitman, R., Sanders, K.M., Zusman, R.M., Healy, A.R., Cheema. F., Lasko, N.B., et al. (2002). Pilot study of secondary prevention of posttraumatic stress disorder with propranolol. *Biol Psychiatry, 51*, 189–192.

259. Taylor, F., & Cahill, L. (2002). Propranolol for reemergent post-traumatic stress disorder following an event of retraumatization: A case study. *J Traumatic Stress, 15*, 433–437.

260. Guillaume, V., Francois, D., Karine, J., Benoit, A., Philippe, L., Alain, B., et al. (in press). Immediate treatment with propranolol decreases PTSD two months after trauma. *Biol Psychiatry.*

261. Holbrook, T. L., Galarneau, M. R., Dye, J. L., Quinn, K., and Dougherty, A. L. (2010). Morphine use after combat injury in Iraq and post-traumatic stress disorder. *New England Journal of Medicine, 362*(2):110–117.

262. Brymer, M.J., Steinberg, A.M., Vernberg, E.M., Layne, C.M., Watson, P.J., Jacobs, A.K., et al. (2009). Acute interventions for children and adolescents. In E.B. Foa, T.M. Keane, M.J. Friedman, & J.A. Cohen (Eds.), *Effective treatments for PTSD: Practice guidelines from the International Society for Traumatic Stress Studies* (2nd ed., pp. 106–116). New York: Guilford.

263. Cohen, J.A. (2003). Treating acute posttraumatic reactions in children and adolescents. *Biol Psychiatry, 53*, 827–833.

264. Robert, R., Blakeney, P.E., Villarreal, C., Rosenberg, L., & Meyer, W.J. 3rd (1999). Imipramine treatment in pediatric burn patients with symptoms of acute stress disorder: A pilot study. *J Am Acad Child Adolesc Psychiatry, 38*, 873–882.

265. Robert, R., Tcheung, W. J., Rosenberg, L., Rosenberg, M., Mitchell, C., Villarreal, C., et al., (2008). Treating thermally injured children suffering symptoms of acute stress with imipramine and fluoxetine: A randomized, double-blind study. *Burns, 34*(7), 919–928.

266. Saxe, G., Stoddar, F., Courtney, D., Cunningham, K., Chawla, N., Sheridan, R., et al. (2001). Relationship between acute morphine and the course of PTSD in children with burns. *J Am Child Adolesc Psychiatry, 40*, 915–921.

267. Prins, A., Ouimette, P., Kimerling, R., Cameron, R.P., Hugeishofer, D.S., Shaw-Hegwer, J., et al. (2004). The primary care PTSD screen (PC-PTSD): Development and operating characteristics. *Primary Care Psychiatry, 9,* 9–14.

268. Brewin, C.R., Rose, S., Andrews, B., Green, J., Tata, P., McEvedy, C., et al. (2002). Brief screening instrument for post-traumatic stress disorder. *British Journal of Psychiatry, 181,* 158–162.

269. Gore, K.L., Engel, C.C., Freed, M.C., Liu, X., & Armsgtrong, D.W. (2008). Test of a single-item posttraumatic stress disorder screener in a military primary care setting. *General Hospital Psychiatry, 30,* 391–397.

270. Norris, F. (1992). Epidemiology of trauma: Frequency and impact of different potentially traumatic events on different demographic groups. *Journal of Consulting and Clinical Psychology, 60*, 409–418.

271. Kilpatrick, D., Resnick, H., & Freedy, J. (1991). *The Potential Stressful Events Interview*. Unpublished instrument, Medical University of South Carolina, Charleston, South Carolina.

272. Vrana, S., & Lauterbach, D. (1994). Prevalence of traumatic events and post-traumatic psychological symptoms in a nonclinical sample of college students. *Journal of Traumatic Stress, 7*, 289–302.

273. Krinsley, K.E., & Weathers, F.W. (1995). The assessment of trauma in adults. *PTSD Research Quarterly, 6*, 1–6.

274. Green, B.L. (1996). Trauma History Questionnaire. In B.H. Stamm & E.M. Varra (Eds.), *Measurement of stress, trauma, and adaptation* (pp. 366–368). Lutherville, MD: Sidran Press.

275. Kubany, E., Haynes, S., Leisen, M., Owens, J., Kaplan, A., Watson, S., et al. (2000). Development and preliminary validation of a brief broad-spectrum measure of trauma exposure: The Traumatic Life Events Questionnaire. *Psychological Assessment, 12*, 210–224.

276. Goodman, L., Corcoran, C., Turner, K., Yuan, N., & Green, B. (1998). Assessing traumatic event exposure: General issues and preliminary findings for the Stressful Life Events Screening Questionnaire. *Journal of Traumatic Stress, 11*, 521–542.

277. Wolfe, J., Kimerling, R., Brown, P.J., Chrestman, K.R., & Levin, K. (1996). Psychometric review of the Life Stressor Checklist-Revised. In B.H. Stamm & E.M. Varra (Eds.), *Measurement of stress, trauma, and adaptation* (pp. 198–201). Lutherville, MD: Sidran Press.

278. Sanders, B., & Becker-Lausen, E. (1995). The measurement of psychological maltreatment: Early data on the Child Abuse and Trauma Scale. *Child Abuse & Neglect, 19*, 315–323.

279. Bernstein, D.P., Fink, L., Handelsman, L. et al. (1994). Initial reliability and validity of a new retrospective measure of child abuse and neglect. *American Journal of Psychiatry, 151*, 1132–1136.

280. Ogata, S.N., Silk, K.R., Goodrich, S., Lohr, N.E., Westen, D., & Hill, E.M. (1990). Childhood sexual and physical abuse in adult patients with borderline personality disorder. *American Journal of Psychiatry, 147*, 1008–1013.

281. Gallagher, R.E., Flye, B.L., Hurt, S.W., Stone, M.H., & Hull, J.W. (1992). Retrospective assessment of traumatic experiences (RATE). *Journal of Personality Disorders, 6*, 99–108.

282. Bremner, J.D., Randall, P., Scott, T.M., Capelli, S., Delany, R., McCarthy, G., et al. (1995). Deficits in short-term memory in adult survivors of childhood abuse. *Psychiatry Research, 59*, 97–107.

283. Straus, M. (1979). Measuring intrafamily conflict and violence: The Conflict Tactics (CT) Scales. *Journal of Marriage and the Family, 41*, 75–88.

284. Shepard, M.F., & Campbell, J.A. (1992). The Abusive Behavior Inventory: A measure of psychological and physical abuse. *Journal of Interpersonal Violence, 7*, 291–305.

285. Koss, M.P., & Gidycz, C.A. (1985). Sexual experiences survey: Reliability and validity. *Journal of Consulting and Clinical Psychology, 53*, 422–423.

286. Wyatt, G.E., Lawrence, J., Vodounon, A., & Mickey, M.R. (1992). The Wyatt Sex History Questionnaire: A structured interview for female sexual history taking. *Journal of Child Sexual Abuse, 1*(4), 51–68.

287. Keane, T.M., Fairbank, J.A., Caddell, J.M., Zimering, R.T., Taylor, K.L., & Mora, C.A. (1989). Clinical evaluation of a measure to assess combat exposure. *Psychological Assessment, 1*, 53–55.

288. Wolfe, J., Brown, P.J., Furey, J., & Levin, K.B. (1993). Development of a wartime stressor scale for women. *Psychological Assessment, 5,* 330–335.

289. Mollica, R.F., Caspi-Yavin, Y., Bollini, P., Truong, T., Tor, S., & Lavelle, J. (1992). The Harvard Trauma Questionnaire: Validating a cross-cultural instrument for measuring torture, trauma, and posttraumatic stress disorder in Indochinese refugees. *Journal of Nervous and Mental Disease, 180,* 111–116.

290. First, MB, Spitzer, R.L., Williams, J.B.W., & Gibbon, M. (1996). *Structured Clinical Interview for DSM-IV.* New York: New York State Psychiatric Institute, Biometrics Research.

291. Blake, D.D., Weathers, F.W., Nagy, L.M., Kaloupek, D.G., Gusman, F.D., Charney, D.S., et al. (1995). The development of a clinician-administered PTSD scale. *Journal of Traumatic Stress, 8,* 75–90.

292. Foa, E., Riggs, D., Dancu, C., & Rothbaum, B. (1993). Reliability and validity of a brief instrument for assessing post-traumatic stress disorder. *Journal of Traumatic Stress, 6,* 459–474.

293. Davidson, J.R.T., Smith, R.D., & Kudler, H.S. (1989). Validity and reliability of the DSM-III criteria for post-traumatic stress disorder: Experience with a structured interview. *Journal of Nervous and Mental Disease,* 177, 336–341.

294. DiNardo, P.A., Brown, T.A., & Barlow, D.H. (1994). *Anxiety Disorders Interview Schedule for DSM-IV: Lifetime Version, (ADIS-IV-L).* San Antonio, TX: Psychological Corporation.

295. Watson, C., Juba, M., Manifold, V., Kucala, T., & Anderson, P. (1991). The PTSD Interview: Rationale, description, reliability and concurrent validity of a DSM-III based technique. *Journal of Clinical Psychology, 47,* 179–185.

296. World Health Organization. (1997). *Composite International Diagnostic Interview (CIDI),* Version 2.1. Geneva: World Health Organization.

297. Robins, L.M., Cottler, L., & Bucholz, K. (1995). *Diagnostic Interview Schedule for DSM-IV.* St Louis: Washington University.

298. Weathers, F.W., Litz, B.T., Herman, D.S., Huska, J.A., & Keane, T.M. (1995). *PTSD Checklist (PCL).* Boston: National Center for PTSD.

299. Foa, E., Cashman, L., Jaycox, L., & Perry, K. (1997). The validation of a self-report measure of posttraumatic stress disorder. *Psychological Assessment, 9,* 445–451.

300. Davidson, J.R.T., Book, S.W., Colket, J.T., Tupler, L.A., Roth, S., David, D., et al. (1997). Assessment of a new self-rating scale for post-traumatic stress disorder. *Psychological Medicine, 27,* 153–160.

301. Briere, J. (2001), *Detailed assessment of adult posttraumatic states: Phenomenology, diagnosis and measurement* (2nd ed.). Washington, D.C., American Psychological Association.

302. Weiss, D.S., & Marmar, C.R. (1997). The Impact of Event Scale—Revised. In J.P. Wilson & T.M. Keane (Eds.), *Assessing psychological trauma and PTSD* (pp. 399–411). London: Guilford Press.

303. Keane, T.M., Caddell, J.M., & Taylor, K.L. (1988). Mississippi Scale for Combat-Related Posttraumatic Stress Disorder: Three studies in reliability and validity. *Journal of Consulting and Clinical Psychology, 56,* 85–90.

304. Lyons, J., & Keane, T. (1992). Keane PTSD Scale: MMPI and MMPI-2 update. *Journal of Traumatic Stress, 5,* 111–117.

305. Briere, J., & Runtz, M. (1989). The Trauma Symptom Checklist (TSC-33): Early data on a new scale. *Journal of Interpersonal Violence, 4*, 151–163.

306. Briere, J. (1995). *Trauma Symptom Inventory (TSI): Professional manual*. Odessa, FL: Psychological Assessment Resources.

307. Hammarberg, M. (1992). Penn Inventory for Posttraumatic Stress Disorder: Psychometric properties. *Psychological Assessment, 4*, 67–76.

308. Kubany, E.S., Leien, M.B., Kaplan, A.S., & Kelly, M.P., (2000), Validation of a brief measure of posttraumatic stress disorder: The Distressing Event Questionnaire. *Psychological Assessment, 12*, 197–209.

309. National Center for Study of Corporal Punishment and Alternatives in Schools. (1992). *My Worst Experience Survey*. Philadelphia, PA: Temple University Press.

310. Ribbe, D. (1996). Psychometric review of Traumatic Event Screening Instrument for Children (TESI-C). In Stamm, B.H. (Ed.), *Measurement of stress, trauma and adaptation* (pp. 386–387). Lutherville, MD: Sidran Press.

311. Fletcher, K. (1991). *When Bad Things Happen Scale*. (Available from the author, University of Massachusetts Medical Center, Dept. of Psychiatry, 55 Lake Avenue North, Worcester, MA 01655.)

312. Friedrich, W. (1995). Evaluation and treatment: The clinical use of the Child Sexual Behavior Inventory: Commonly asked questions. *American Professional Society on the Abuse of Children (APSAC) Advisor, 8*(1), 17–20.

313. Praver, F. (1994). *Child Rating Scales—Exposure to Interpersonal Abuse*. Unpublished copyrighted instrument.

314. Praver, F., Pelcovitz, D., & DiGiuseppe, R. (1994). *The Angie/Andy Child Rating Scales* (Available from Praver, 5 Marseilles Drive, Locust Valley, NY 11560; Pelcovitz, Dept. of Psychiatry, 400 Community Drive, Manhasset, NY 11030; or DiGiuseppe, Psychology Dept., St. John's University, Grand Central and Utopia Parkways, Jamaica, NY 11439.)

315. Reich, W., Leacock, N., & Shanfield, C. (1994). *Diagnostic Interview for Children and Adolescents-Revised (DICA-R)*. St. Louis, MO: Washington University.

316. Newman, W., Weathers, F.W., Nader, K., Kaloupek, D.G., Pynoos, R.S., Blake, D.D., et al. (2004). *Clinician-Administered PTSD Scale for Children and Adolescents(Caps-CA)*. Los Angeles: Western Psychological Services.

317. Shaffer, D., Fisher, P., Lucas, C.P., Dulcan, M., & Schwab-Stone, M. (2000). The NIMH Diagnostic Interview Schedule for Children, Version IV (DISC-IV): Description, differences from previous versions and reliability of some common diagnoses. *Journal of the American Academy of Child and Adolescent Psychiatry*, 39, 28–38.

318. Yasik,A.E., Saigh,P.A., Oberfield, R.A., Green, B.L., & McHugh, M. (2001). The validity of the Children's PTSD Inventory. *Journal of Traumatic Stress, 14*, 81–94.

319. Pynoos, R.S., Rodriguez, N., Sternberg, A. Stauber, M. & Frederick, C. (1998). *UCLA PTSD Index for DSM-V-Child Version*. Los Angeles, UCLA Trauma Psychiatry Service.

320. Kaufman, J., Birmaher, B., Brent, D., Rao, U., Flynn, C., Moreci, P., et al. (1997). Schedule for Affective Disorder and Schizophrenia for

School-Age Children—Present and Lifetime Version (K-SADS-PL): Initial reliability and validity data. *Journal of the American Academy of Child and Adolescent Psychiatry,* 36, 980–988.

321. Scheeringa, M.S., & Zeanah, C.H. (1994). *PTSD Semi-Structured Interview and Observational Record for Infants and Young Children.* New Orleans: Department of Psychiatry and Neurology, Tulane University Health Sciences Center.

322. Ahmad, A., Sundelin-Wahlsten, V., Sofi, M.A., Qahar, J.A., & von Knorring, A.L. (2000). Reliability and validity of a child-specific cross-cultural instrument for assessing posttraumatic stress disorder. *European Child and Adolescent Psychiatry. 9,* 285–294.

323. Briere, J. (1996a). *Trauma Symptom Checklist for Children (TSCC).* Odessa, FL: Psychological Assessment Resources.

324. Briere, J. (1996b). *Trauma Symptom Checklist for Children (TSCC) professional manual.* Odessa, FL: Psychological Assessment Resources.

325. Foa, E.B., Johnson, K.M., Feeny, N.C., & Treadwell, K.R. (2001). The Child PTSD Symptom Scale: A preliminary examination of its psychometric properties. *Journal of Clinical Child Psychology, 30,* 376–384.

326. Greenwald, R. (2000). *Child Report of Post-Traumatic Symptoms (CROPS) and Parent Report of Post-Traumatic Symptoms (PROPS): Manual and measures.* Baltimore, MD: Sidran.

327. Levandosky, A.A., Huth-Boks, A.C., Semel, M.A., & Shapiro, D.L. (2002). Trauma symptoms in pre-school-age children exposed to domestic violence. *Journal of Interpersonal Violence.* 17, 150–164.

328. Achenbach, T.M., & Rescoria, L. (2000). *Child Behavior Checklist for Ages 1½–5.* Burlington, University of Vermont.

Index

Note: Italicized page locators indicate a figure.